MOTHER MASSAGE

MOTHER MASSAGE

*A Handbook
for Relieving the
Discomforts of Pregnancy*

ELAINE STILLERMAN, LMT

Illustrations by Diana Kurz

A DELL TRADE PAPERBACK

A DELL TRADE PAPERBACK

Published by
Dell Publishing
a division of
Bantam Doubleday Dell Publishing Group, Inc.
1540 Broadway
New York, New York 10036

Library of Congress Cataloging in Publication Data
Stillerman, Elaine.
    Mother Massage: a handbook for relieving the discomforts of pregnancy/Elaine Stillerman; illustrations by Diana Kurz.
      p. cm.
    ISBN 0-440-50702-2
    1. Prenatal care. 2. Massage. 3. Pregnancy. 4. Childbirth.
5. Postnatal care. I. Title.
RG525.S695 1992
618.2'4—dc20   91-46989 CIP

Manufactured in the United States of America

Published simultaneously in Canada

August 1992

10 9 8 7 6

RRH

*This book is lovingly dedicated
to Robert and Kaye.*

ACKNOWLEDGMENTS

This book would not have been possible without the help and support of all the expectant couples I have worked with. Special thanks go to Alice Brown, Bob Yoder, Jacalyn Barnett, and Madeleine Morel.

Elaine Stillerman, a licensed massage therapist in New York City, has been specializing in prenatal and postpartum massage since 1980 and has worked with hundreds of expectant women. She has written many articles on massage therapy and teaches the nationally certified course "MotherMassage: Massage During Pregnancy" at massage schools all over the country. She is also the author of *The Encyclopedia of Bodywork* (1996).

CONTENTS

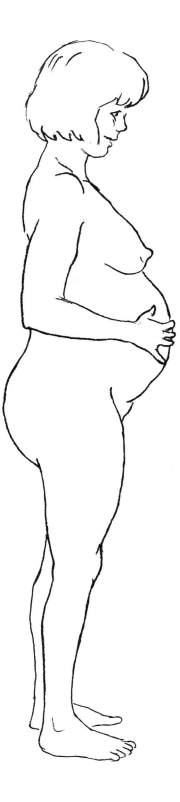

PREFACE

*D*uring pregnancy, women suffer from all sorts of ailments, including heartburn, backaches, swollen ankles, aching muscles, breast soreness, and fatigue, to mention just a few. Traditional medicine offers few means of alleviating these problems. In addition, women may feel increased stress due to the psychological effects of pregnancy, which include changes in body image, concerns about the baby's health, motherhood, and the challenge of this life-changing event.

Mother Massage can help. In this groundbreaking book, you will discover the power of a therapeutic and loving touch. You will learn how truly to share the joy and excitement of your pregnancy with your partner. And you will explore the many ways of relieving the discomforts of pregnancy through massage.

Through simple techniques, including the nerve stroke, effleurage, petrissage, friction, and tapotement, a wide range of treatments can be mastered and shared. You will learn how massage can relieve tension during pregnancy, help prepare you for labor, and make the postpartum period less difficult. *Mother Massage* includes valuable advice on reflexology, nutrition, herbology, and exercise, as well as a special section on baby massage.

This book is lovingly written. I have seen the techniques work with my wife and myself. I am pleased to recommend this to every parent who is bringing a new life into the world.

RONALD RUDEN, M.D.
Lenox Hill Hospital
New York, N.Y.

INTRODUCTION

*M*uch has been written and scientifically validated about the beneficial effects of massage on almost every major body system. It is also a well-documented fact that massage is a powerful tool in reducing stress and its deleterious effects.

The stress and anxiety a pregnant woman experiences will definitely work against her: Blood catecholamine[1] levels increase and interfere with the work of oxytocin and other labor-promoting hormones. There is also an adverse effect on the developing fetus. In other words, whatever the expectant mother feels is directly passed on to her growing child.

Enter the oldest healing art: massage. During pregnancy, massage can safely, comfortably, and effectively relieve stress, whether it is physical, emotional, and/or psychological in origin. With so many women returning to more holistic health choices and birthing practices, the use of massage to treat the discomforts of pregnancy is a natural response. Massage is a potent way to take charge of your own pregnancy, to reclaim your birthright. Every time you experience a positive response to the treatments in this book, your success empowers you with more control, security, and confidence for an easier birth outcome.

---

1. Catecholamines are compounds responsible for the "fight or flight" response to stress.

Mother Massage has been written to involve both expectant parents. Fathers now share birth preparation classes, attend the births, and are more aggressively pursuing paternity rights and privileges in the workplace. By using the easy massage techniques in this book, he can also participate during the nine-month process and help support and ease the discomforts of his partner's pregnancy.

Each technique is no longer than ten or fifteen minutes in duration and is clearly illustrated for easy reference. The treatments reduce the effects of many of the most common problems a pregnant woman might incur and can be used as often as necessary.

The intimate nature of touch has the additional advantage of bringing two people closer together. At a time when emotions and sensitivities are already heightened, massage enhances interpersonal communication even further. A deeper involvement develops for the provider as he helps his partner enjoy this most exciting experience.

Infant massage is included as a natural progression to the pregnancy. This special treatment helps both child and parent form a unique bond of love, trust, and nurturing. It also offers the father an opportunity to express his tender feelings, no longer considered an exclusive maternal right.

All attempts have been made to clarify when each partner is being addressed. *Mother Massage* speaks to the expectant mother about the development of her pregnancy and self-massage techniques. The expectant father is addressed during most of the massage techniques of Chapter 2 (Chapter 3 is for both partners equally), labor, and postpartum massages.

My expectant clients respond to their pregnancies with the most interesting reactions. Some of them are astounded how their bodies know just what to do. Others have to be reassured that pregnancy is not a permanent condition and that their figures will return. Most of them agree, however, about how strong, ready, and prepared they feel as a result of the massages.

Use *Mother Massage* throughout your pregnancy and postpartum weeks. The chapter on full body massage can be used at any time after the pregnancy and for either partner. So I hope you enjoy this book and reap the benefits of massage for a long time!

ELAINE STILLERMAN
New York City, 1991

MOTHER MASSAGE

CHAPTER 1

THE MASSAGE TECHNIQUES

Women in tribal societies resume normal activities almost immediately after birthing. To get back into shape quickly, these women employ a number of natural techniques, including massage, abdominal binding, herbal treatments, diet, and steaming of the perineal region. All of these methods help the new mother to regain her strength, heal faster, and ease her way in subsequent births.

Massage is a sensuous, relaxing, and loving treatment that has the added bonus of being especially good for you. It is one form of "medicine" most people delight in taking! Massage is a wonderful way to reduce stress and promote general well-being.

While you are pregnant, your body is undergoing stress-producing changes. Massage pleasantly and effectively eliminates many of the adverse effects of stress and the accompanying discomforts. Let's look briefly at some of the physiological changes that occur during a massage and see how they benefit your health and the health of your developing baby:

• Massage will help prepare you for an easier delivery. Self-massage to the perineum (the area between the vagina and anus) promotes flexibility and elasticity. It might actually help you avoid an episiotomy.

• Massage stimulates glandular secretions, stabilizing your hormonal levels and making their side effects less severe.

• Massage to the legs can control varicose veins, and the draining effect of massage facilitates reduction of edema (swelling) of the extremities.

• An increase in general circulation offers a rise of blood to all areas of your body, including the placenta. This brings greater nutrition to the tissues of the body and enhances waste product removal.

• "Lazy" red blood cells lining the vessel walls are reintroduced into circulation, thus increasing the red blood cell count. This is of particular importance to those women with anemia. A rise in the red blood cell count also helps to eliminate fatigue, since more oxygen-carrying hemoglobin is released into the bloodstream.

• The lymphatic system circulates faster and more efficiently. The result is more energy and less fatigue.

• The strain on the muscles of the lower back, abdomen, and shoulders can be greatly reduced through massage. As your pregnancy advances to its final trimester, this relief will be most welcome.

• Muscle tone can increase with regular massage. Muscle spasms and knots are easily released, and muscles, ligaments, tendons, and joints enjoy greater flexibility. This is most advantageous during labor.

• Massage sedates the nervous system, producing much-needed rest and relaxation. In utero, your baby feels the same way. Frazzled nerves are lovingly soothed, and insomnia can be relieved.

Massage accompanies childbirth nearly everywhere in the tribal world. Noted anthropologist George Englemann, who studied tribal customs, wrote in 1884, "There is hardly a people, ancient or modern, that do not in some way resort to massage and expression in labor, even if it be a natural and easy one."[1] The elder women of the Nama Hottentot tribe of South Africa massage the expectant mothers several times a week in preparation for childbirth. Pregnant women of Uganda receive treatment to make their bones supple for an easy delivery. Women of Kiribati (formerly the Gilbert Islands) receive "shampoos" by expert massage practitioners to train their muscles to bear contractions.

The massage techniques you will be using are derived from Swedish massage, Shiatsu acupressure, and foot reflexology. *Mother Massage* also includes herbal remedies, nutritional information, and exercises and postures as part of its holistic scope of pregnancy health care.

The Swedish strokes are effleurage, petrissage, friction, tapotement, and the nerve stroke.

EFFLEURAGE

Effleurage is the stroke you will begin and end each treatment with. This long, gliding movement introduces the massage and prepares the muscles for deeper work. This movement is primarily responsible for the increase in circulation of blood and lymph. It can eliminate fatigue from the body by improving waste removal and increase nutrition to those tissues being treated. You can easily see how important this stroke is to help the expectant woman overcome fatigue. Effleurage is also one of the most pleasurable and sensuous strokes. In the illustrations, effleurage is indicated with short, straight arrows.

PETRISSAGE

Petrissage is popularly referred to as kneading. It applies to any movement that moves muscles over bones and consists of knead-

1. Judith Goldsmith, *Childbirth Wisdom* (New York: Congdon & Weed, 1984), p. 39.

ing, pressing, rolling, and squeezing. Petrissage is responsible for the increase in size and strength of a muscle. For mother's massage, you will use it to increase the tone of weakened and strained muscles. Petrissage, or circular kneading, is indicated with curved arrows.

FRICTION

Friction is generally used in therapeutic treatments to relieve muscle spasms and tension. It is either a circular movement applied to a joint to help restore range of motion and flexibility of the joint, or transversely across the belly of a muscle. The latter application breaks down muscle spasms and is of great importance in the treatment of sciatica.

TAPOTEMENT

Tapotement is also called percussion, and you perform it as if you were playing a drum with hands or fingertips rapidly following each other. It is a stimulatory stroke that can promote muscular contraction, increase the blood supply to a particular area, and enhance nerve response.

NERVE STROKE

The nerve stroke is a very light, gentle fingertip glide down any part of the body. Its purpose is to signal the end of a massage sequence and to sedate all the nerve endings that have been stimulated.

ACUPRESSURE

Acupressure is the basis of the Shiatsu technique. Pressing into a specific point along the energy meridian (channel) will help break up energy blocks, reduce muscular adhesions, increase circulation to a particular area, and produce a relaxed sense of well-being.

FOOT REFLEXOLOGY

This ancient healing art is applied to the feet. Each part of the body has a corresponding point on the foot. Pressing these points offers relief from the discomforts of pregnancy and promotes more energy and better health.

HERBAL REMEDIES

The teas and herbs mentioned in this book are predominantly emmenagogues—that is, they relate to the female reproductive system. They are nontoxic. Many recipes, such as for red raspberry leaf tea, can be taken daily to help tone and strengthen your uterus. The dosage and frequency are given for each recipe. One word of caution: Herbs and other natural remedies should never be taken at the same time as conventional prescribed medications and should not be randomly self-administered without the knowledge of your health care provider or physician.

NUTRITION

Good nutrition during pregnancy is a matter of knowing how much to eat and exactly which foods you need to support yourself and your healthy baby. Some discomforts of pregnancy can be caused by nutritional deficiencies such as anemia; whenever possible, you will be guided to specific foods that may resolve those problems. Appendix II lists USRDA during pregnancy and lactation to help you plan adequate meals for yourself and your family.

EXERCISES AND POSTURES

Many of the problems that arise during pregnancy are due to muscle strain, weakness, and poor posture. The simple exercises are included to help you relieve these aches and complaints. Proper exercise will increase your energy, strengthen the muscles most strained during pregnancy and labor, stimulate circulation, increase flexibility in the joints, and control swelling in the extremities.

One of the best overall workouts is swimming. It places no stress on the joints and is an efficient aerobic exercise and toner. Walking or cycling are also wonderful activities that are safe for pregnant women. Weight training is becoming popular to give added muscle tone and strength in preparation for childbirth. Many exercise classes are specially designed for pregnant women. These classes are very beneficial in controlling weight gain and maintaining muscle tone.

Exercise also has the advantage of providing the pregnant woman with a sense of control over her ever-changing body, and it boosts her ofttimes fragile self-image.

Consult with your physician or health care provider before beginning any program of exercise.

CONTRAINDICATIONS OF MASSAGE

There are times during your pregnancy when you should *not* receive a massage. These contraindications are:

- when you have morning sickness, nausea, or vomiting

- with any vaginal bleeding or discharge

- when you have a fever

- when you notice a decrease in fetal movement over a twenty-four-hour period

- when you have diarrhea

- if you experience pain in the abdomen or anywhere else in your body

- if you notice excessive swelling in your arms or legs

- do not massage directly on top of a bruise or skin irritation; this includes direct massage to keloid scars, those thick, red, ropy scars that might have resulted from a previous C-section or other surgical procedure

- do not massage immediately after eating; wait at least two hours

- if your doctor or health care provider disapproves for any other medical reason

SUPPLIES

You don't need a lot of equipment to make the massage a pleasurable experience. However, you will need:

- a warm room free from drafts, breezes, and noise

- some sort of cushioning for the floor, such as a sleeping bag, mat, or blanket

- sheets to protect the cushion and the furniture when you will be massaged in a seated position

- extra towels

- extra pillows; one will be for the massage provider

- massage oil; vegetable oil is fine—remember to put the oil in a plastic bottle to avoid breakage

- moisturizing creams or lotions for the face if preferred over oil

- clean hands and short fingernails

- music and candlelight to enhance the mood

CHAPTER 2

RELIEVING THE DISCOMFORTS OF PREGNANCY

*D*uring pregnancy, the changes in a woman's body and natural fears and anxieties are all stress-producing. General massage is one of the most efficient, pleasant, and sensuous ways to reduce stress and its detrimental side effects. However, the more common complaints that occur during pregnancy can also be easily and comfortably alleviated through use of the following massage techniques.

These techniques are based on years of research and application and are built on the principles that you can take charge of your own pregnancy and that your partner can participate in this exciting experience. Listed in alphabetical order for easy reference, these common discomforts are treated naturally through massage, reflexology, herbs, nutrition, and simple exercises and postures.

It is wonderful to know that you can help yourself, and be helped, during your pregnancy. Every time you successfully react to a treatment, you are learning to control your body. As labor draws nearer, your experiences will reinforce a positive reaction to the birthing process. These techniques will help ease many of your discomforts, thereby allowing you to enjoy this miraculous experience of childbearing.

9

ABDOMINAL PRESSURE

The following techniques will also help relieve constipation, gas, and heartburn.

As the baby grows, so does the pressure on the organs and tissues of the abdomen. This pressure can be uncomfortable, but exercises that relax and strengthen the muscles of the abdomen will help ease a lot of this discomfort. It also helps to keep the bladder and intestines empty whenever possible.

1. **Pelvic tilt** (see illustration 2.1)

- Lie on the floor, knees bent, feet pulled up to the buttocks. Put your arms at your sides or crossed over your abdomen.
- Slowly lift from the buttocks up the spine to the maximum tilt. Keep your feet flat on the floor.
- Hold the position for five to ten seconds. Breathe normally.
- Slowly return to the original position, lowering the upper back first, down the spine to the small of your back. Take a deep breath. Exhale. Repeat four more times.

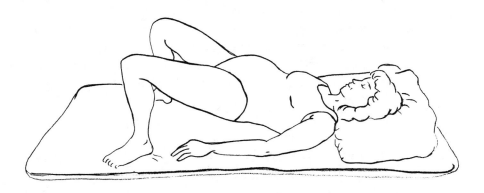

2.1 ————————————————————————————————————

Pelvic tilt for relief of abdominal pressure, gas, and constipation.

2. Four-point pelvic tilt (also helps relieve lower back pain) (see illustration 2.2)

- Kneel on your hands and knees, keeping your back straight. Inhale.
- Exhale and round out the lower back, bringing your chin to your chest at the same time. Hold to a count of five.
- Inhale and return to the original position. Do not let your back sway in this position. Repeat four more times.

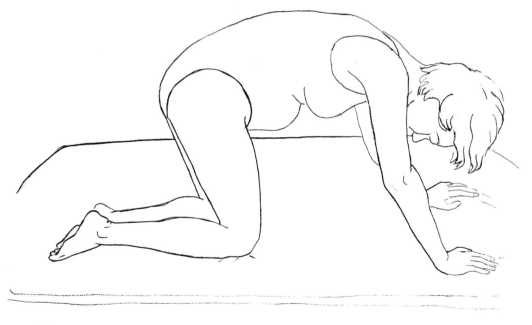

2.2

Four-point pelvic tilt for relief of abdominal pressure, lower back pain, gas, and constipation.

3. Knee-chest rest (see illustration 2.3)

- Kneel on slightly spread knees.
- Bend over. Place an ear on the floor. Bring both arms to rest on the floor next to your legs.
- Breathe normally. Stay like this for one full minute, then turn your head to the other side for another minute.

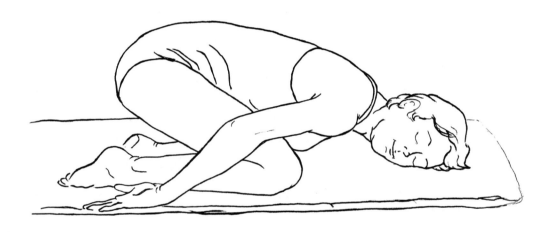

2.3

Knee-chest rest for relief of abdominal pressure, gas, and constipation.

ALLERGIES AND SINUS CONGESTION

Even if you have never suffered from allergies before, pregnancy can create stuffiness and nasal congestion caused by swollen mucous membranes, or sinus headaches brought on by dry nasal passages. Dairy foods increase production of mucus, so it is advisable to limit yourself to skim milk products and get your calcium through additional sources.

These foods include dry nonfat milk powder; salmon with bones; sardines with bones; soybeans and soy products such as tofu; Brazil nuts, hazelnuts, and almonds; ground sesame seeds; seaweed (dulse, wakame, amanori, or hijiki found in health food stores or Oriental markets); legumes such as black beans, chickpeas (garbanzo beans), and pinto beans; and dark, leafy green vegetables such as collard greens, dandelion greens, spinach, turnip greens, okra, and broccoli.

It is advisable to avoid foods to which you are allergic; also, stay away from smoke-filled rooms to reduce irritation to the nasal passages.

H I N T S : Inhale steam from a vaporizer, a hot shower, or from boiling water. This helps to open and drain stuffed sinuses. Put a few drops of eucalyptus oil in the water to help reduce swelling of the sinus membranes. It also helps to apply a warm, moist towel on your face directly above the sinuses.

M A S S A G E : This technique can be self-administered, or performed by your partner. If you wear contact lenses, removing them will provide greater comfort.

Pressure point massage to the sinuses is very effective in promoting drainage. Hold each point for thirty seconds.

1. Press deeply on the frontal points of the forehead (see illustration 2.4).

2. Press the bridge of the nose with your little fingers (see illustration 2.4).

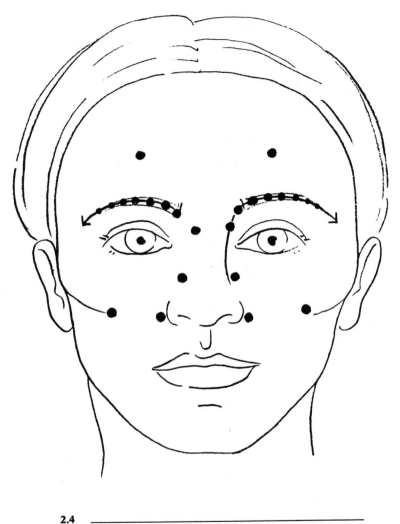

2.4

Pressure points for allergies and sinus congestion.

3. Stretch along the eyebrow ridge.

4. Press the points halfway down the nose.

5. Press in at the points at the nostrils (see illustration 2.4).

6. Press in the center of the cheekbones. Try to hook under the bone (see illustration 2.4).

7. Rub down the nose, fanning out under the cheekbone (see illustration 2.4).

8. Squeeze the muscles at the back of the neck.

R E F L E X O L O G Y : This can also be self-administered, or performed by your partner.

The sinus reflexes are at the fleshy part of the tips of the toes (see illustration 2.5). Hold each point for thirty seconds.

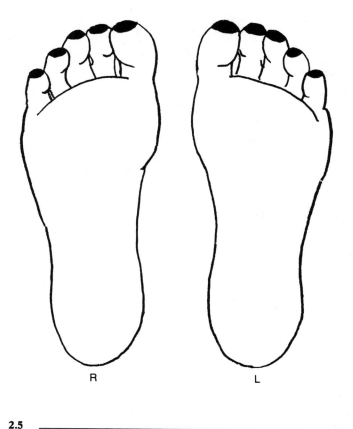

R   L

2.5 _____

Reflex points for relief of allergies and sinus congestion.

ANEMIA

Due to the increased demands placed on the pregnant woman's body, iron deficiency anemia is a very common ailment. It is a condition in which there is an insufficient level of hemoglobin in the blood. Hemoglobin, which gives blood its red color, receives oxygen from the lungs and then delivers it to the cells of the body. Without enough hemoglobin, the entire body, including the developing baby, has a shortage of oxygen.

Symptoms of anemia are fatigue, loss of appetite, brittle nails, lackluster skin, dizziness, and pallor. Since iron produces hemoglobin, the obvious solution is to increase the iron intake, either in the form of a supplement administered by your physician or health care provider or through food sources. It is not unusual to hear that many women who take iron supplements find them constipating.

Dietary sources rich in iron are liver; lean and organ meats; fish; clams and oysters; eggs; whole grains; cream of wheat; wheat germ (two tablespoons); dark, leafy greens such as spinach, beans, dandelion greens, kale, parsley, soybeans, prunes, raisins, apricots, and almonds; and one tablespoon of blackstrap molasses.

Herbs rich in iron are dandelion and yellow dock.

Vitamin C is necessary for proper iron absorption along with calcium. Both these elements increase the body's ability to absorb and use iron. There are other elements, such as oxalates in dark, leafy green vegetables, that bind with iron to form an insoluble compound. Therefore, the iron found in meat or fish is more easily absorbed. Phosphates, chiefly found in soft drinks, also inhibit the body's ability to absorb iron.

MASSAGE: By the partner. A full body massage will reduce the fatigue that accompanies anemia. Massage has long been recognized to increase blood and lymph circulation. Therefore, oxygenated blood, rich in nutrients, is brought to tissue cells, as metabolic waste, and the by-products of tissue damage, are transported from the cells. Stimulated circulation can raise the red blood cell count and thereby produce more hemoglobin. See the chapter on full body massage for a description of this technique.

REFLEXOLOGY: The reflex point for anemia is on the left foot, at the point of the spleen (see illustration 2.6). The spleen recycles iron and plays an important role in the manufacture of hemoglobin. Locate the area on the left foot and press into it until slight pressure is felt. Reflex work can be uncomfortable, so work up to your partner's tolerance level slowly. Hold the point until any tenderness or soreness on that spot disappears.

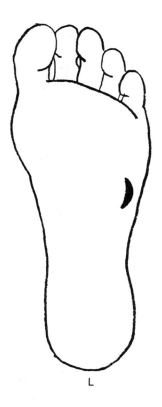

L

2.6

The reflex point for the treatment of anemia is found on the left foot only.

BACKACHES

Backaches rank high in the top ten complaints of pregnancy, especially in the last trimester. Weight displacement, the change in the center of gravity, and the weight gain add up to discomfort and soreness for the muscles of the back.

MASSAGE: By the partner. This can be done lying down or sitting in a chair. In either position, strategically placed pillows offer additional comfort and support. The mother can lean onto a pillow on a table if she is sitting.

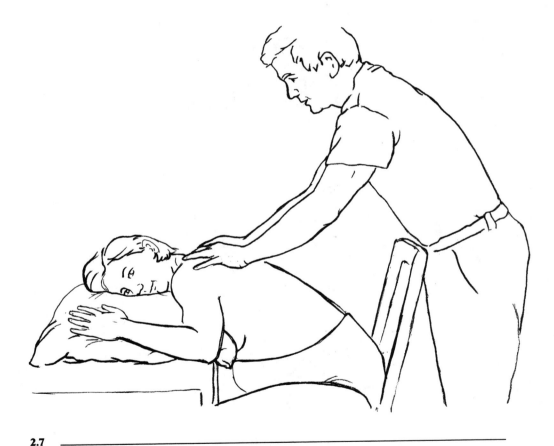

2.7

Effleurage of the upper back in a seated position.

Seated, Upper Back

1. Find a comfortable position, standing behind the mother.

2. Squeeze a small amount of oil on your hands and rub them together vigorously. This will warm the oil. The first stroke of the massage is also the stroke that spreads the lubrication on the mother's back. Effleurage from the middle of her back to the shoulders (see illustration 2.7). Repeat two or three more times to get the oil evenly distributed.

3. Repeat the same stroke with deeper pressure. Circle around each shoulder with one hand.

4. With the thumbs, make small circles all along the border of the shoulder blade (see illustration 2.8). This is an area of sensitive pressure points: If any spot feels particularly good—eliciting a "good hurt" response—stay with it. Keep circling that spot with your thumbs until the soreness dissipates.

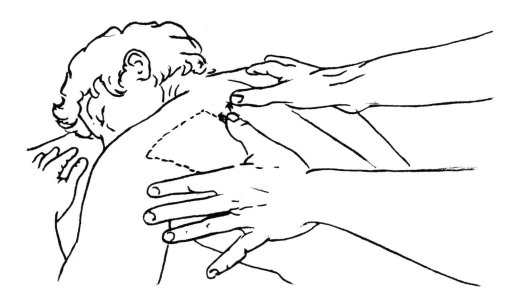

2.8

Circular kneading of the border of the shoulder blade in a seated position.

5. Gently squeeze the top of each shoulder between your palms.

6. Place one hand on her forehead as she drops her head into your hand. With your other hand, rub up and down the back of her neck (see illustration 2.9). Repeat this stroke several times.

7. Return to the shoulders and repeat the first stroke a few more times, from the middle of her back to her shoulders. It's always a good idea to finish a treatment the same way you began it. This signals an end to the massage. You can repeat the strokes that feel particularly good at any time.

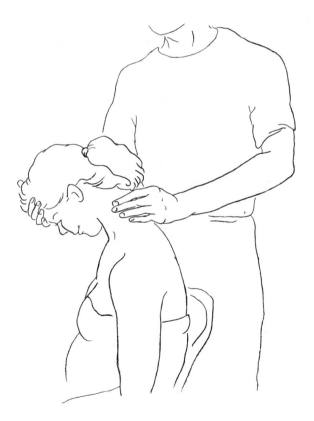

2.9 _____

Neck effleurage in a seated position.

Seated, Lower Back

1. After massaging the upper back, stand to one side of the mother and run one hand all the way up her back on the side of the spine closest to you. Work from the hip to the top of her shoulder with an effleurage stroke (see illustration 2.10). Repeat a few more times, and then repeat on her other side.

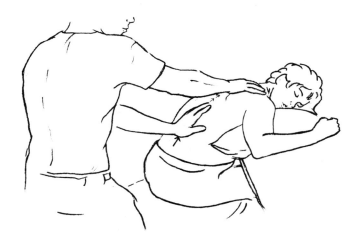

2.10

Effleurage of the back in a seated position.

2. Kneel down behind your partner and place both thumbs on her sacrum (the small triangular bone at the base of the spine). Make small circles, alternating your thumbs, directly on the bone (see illustration 2.11).

3. Repeat the full back stroke, using both of your hands at the same time.

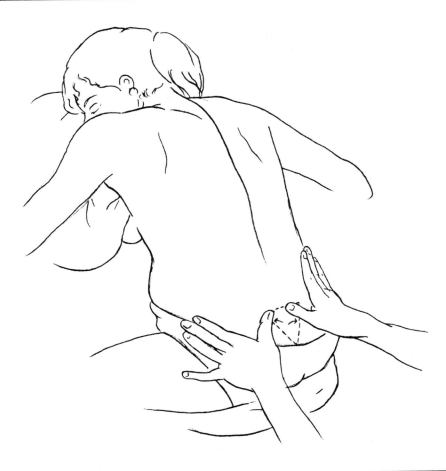

2.11

Alternate thumb kneading on the sacrum.

LYING DOWN: The mother will have to lie on one side and support herself with pillows. One pillow should go under her head, another between her knees. The belly may be supported with a pillow if it makes her more comfortable (see illustration 2.12).

In this position, the massage can be applied to only one side of her back at a time.

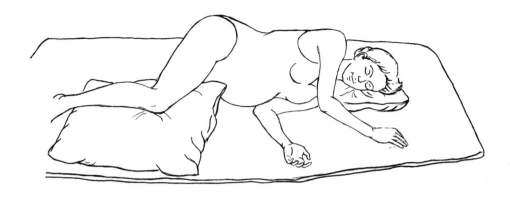

2.12

Side-lying posture showing placement of pillows.

1. Sit behind your partner. Place one hand on top of her shoulder for support. Effleurage from her hip up to and around her shoulder (see illustration 2.13). Repeat this stroke several more times with increased pressure.

2. Circle all around her shoulder. Much of the weight displacement is also felt in the shoulder area, so concentrate on this area by repeating the stroke several more times with increased pressure. Effleurage up and down her neck.

3. Gently squeeze the muscles on the top of the shoulder.

4. With your thumbs, make tiny circles along the border of the shoulder blade (see illustration 2.14). Make a larger circle all around the shoulder as you did before, using an open hand.

5. Once you feel the muscles relax, you can apply more pressure. Keeping one hand on her shoulder, make small circles on the large, ropy muscle directly beside the spine with your fingertips (see illustration 2.14). The pressure is toward the spine. Work from the neck down to the hip, and effleurage from the hip to her neck to compete the movement.

2.13

Effleurage of the back in a side-lying posture.

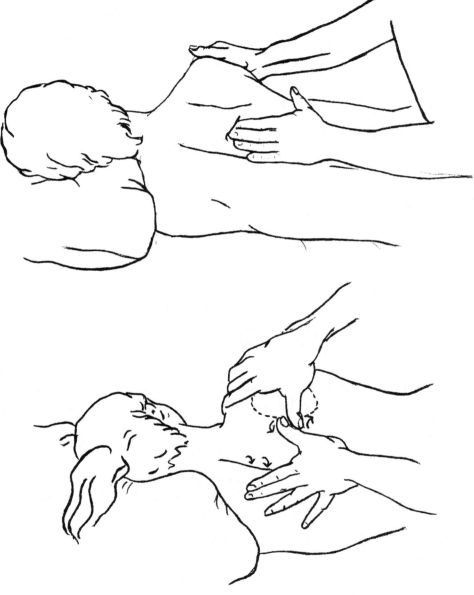

2.14

Circular kneading along the border of the scapula; circular kneading along the spine.

6. When working on the back, you must not overlook the neck or the hips. You can't release the stress in a muscle group without massaging all the muscles in the group. Support your partner at her shoulder, and with the heel of your palm, make a large circle on her buttock. Repeat the same circle on her sacrum (see illustration 2.15).

7. Finish this side with a few more long, fluid effleurage strokes from her hip over her shoulder.

Remove the pillows carefully, and gently help her turn over so you can repeat the same sequence on the other side.

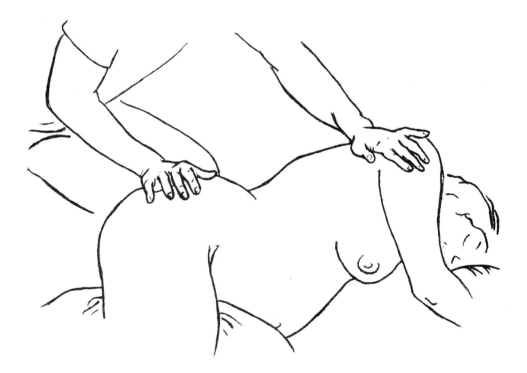

2.15

Large circle on the buttock with heel of the palm.

REFLEXOLOGY: The reflex points for the back vary according to the position on the spine. The neck reflex is on the "neck" of the toes and on the inner part of the big toe (see illustration 2.16a). The midback reflex is on the inner edge of the foot on the arch, midway down the foot, and across the top in the middle (see illustration 2.16b). The lower back area is at the heel. This is a good area to work on if sciatica—the painful inflammation of the sciatic nerve—is a problem.

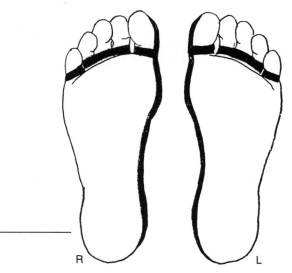

2.16a

Reflex points of the back.

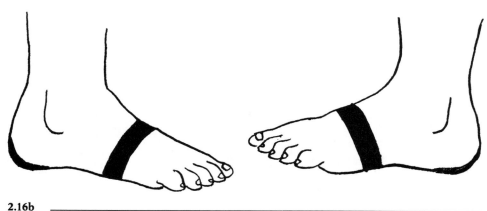

2.16b

Reflex points of the back.

Use your thumb to rub back and forth along these areas. It is generally advisable to massage the entire arch and all related points, even if soreness appears on only one part of the back.

EXERCISES: In addition to those exercises listed in the section for abdominal pressure, other stretches can help relax the muscles of the back.

1. Knee-chest stretch (see illustration 2.17)

- Lie on the floor. Bring one knee to your chest. Breathe.
- Straighten the leg back onto the floor. Flex the other leg, and bring the knee to your chest. Breathe.
- Bring both knees to your chest. Gently rock up and down on the spine. Repeat ten times.

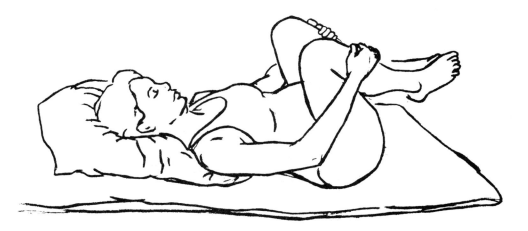

2.17

Knee-chest stretch to relax back muscles.

2. Knee-chest twist (see illustration 2.18)

- Lie on the floor. Pull both knees to your chest.
- Drop your bent knees over to one side. Turn your head and raise your arm in the opposite direction. Breathe normally. Stay like this for thirty to sixty seconds, and then reverse the twist.

H I N T S : Avoid lower back pain by wearing comfortable, low-heeled shoes, and try not to carry heavy objects. Proper body mechanics are especially important now, so when you have to bend down to pick up something, bend your knees and lift with your legs—not your back.

H E R B S : There is a wonderfully aromatic massage oil you can make yourself for use during the back massage or general massage: In two fluid ounces of vegetable oil, add ten drops of juniper, six drops of lavender, and eight drops of rosemary. Use this oil only in the second and third trimesters.

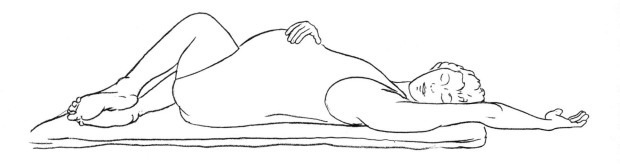

2.18

Knee-chest twist to stretch the muscles of the back.

BREAST SORENESS

Enlarged and tender breasts are usually among the first signs of pregnancy, but much of the initial soreness will subside after the first trimester. However, continued breast enlargement can make them sensitive and unusually heavy. Blood supply increases as the milk glands prepare for lactation, and a network of superficial veins may be visible across the chest. The color of the nipple area will also darken.

Massage to reduce some of the heaviness is a very pleasurable treatment. Don't be alarmed if lactation occurs in the final stages of the pregnancy due to the stimulating effect of the massage and the ensuing release of hormones.

M A S S A G E : This can be self-administered or performed by your partner. Work lightly and carefully, and avoid direct nipple contact.

1. Using oil or cream, lightly circle around both breasts. Keep your pressure light and even.

2. Circle one breast. Using your fingertips, make tiny circles on the breast (see illustration 2.19). You will feel some hardness, maybe even enlarged glands and ducts. Be gentle. Repeat on the other breast.

3. Place both hands flatly on the sides of one breast and slowly slide away from the areola (see illustration 2.20). Change your position around the breast. Do the same movements on the other breast.

H I N T : Wearing a supportive bra will reduce a lot of the breast discomfort you may be feeling. If you are going to nurse your baby, here are a few simple suggestions to toughen your nipples so they won't feel too sore when the baby feeds: Wear a nursing bra, but leave the flaps down to allow your breasts to rub against your blouse; after bathing, rub your nipples with a terry washcloth; some women sunbathe topless to harden their nipples.

2.19

Small fingertip circles to relieve breast soreness.

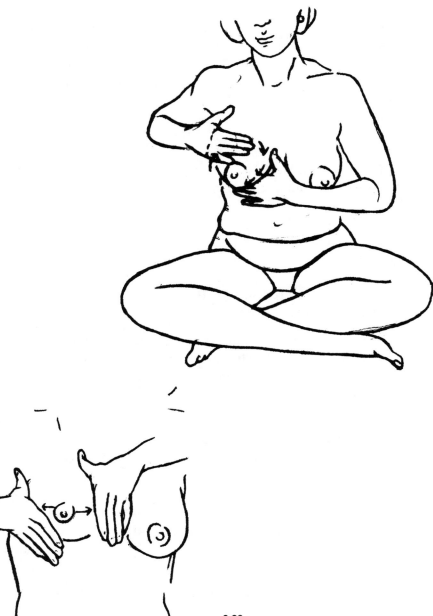

2.20

Slide outward from the areola.

Always apply a lotion after any of these suggestions to avoid dry, cracked skin.

HERBS FOR BREAST SORENESS: Apply a warm ginger compress for thirty minutes. Shave a handful of fresh ginger into simmering water. Let it cook for about fifteen minutes. Take it off the heat and allow the water to cool. Dip a washcloth into the ginger solution and wring out the excess water. Apply the warm compress to your breasts for thirty minutes. Dip the washcloth into the ginger solution every ten minutes.

FOR MASTITIS WHILE NURSING: Mastitis, or breast infection, is not a reason to stop nursing. As a matter of fact, the infection is more easily cured if nursing continues. You don't have

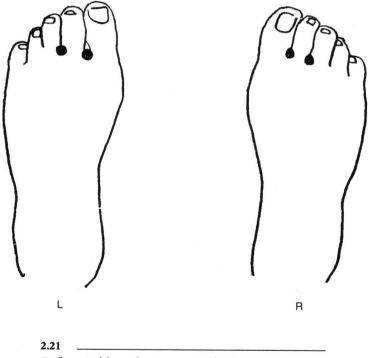

L   R

2.21

Reflex and lymphatic points for breast soreness.

to worry about passing the infection to your baby, since he or she already has the same germs in his or her mouth and nose. Make a warm compress of equal parts of lavender oil, geranium oil, and rose oil in one quart of warm water. Let it cool to a comfortable temperature, and apply the compress to each breast for ten to fifteen minutes.

REFLEXOLOGY:

1. Press the top of the foot between the second and third toes (see illustration 2.21).

2. Press the lymphatic point on the top of the foot between the big and second toes (see illustration 2.21).

CARPAL TUNNEL SYNDROME

Carpal tunnel syndrome (CTS), a painful condition affecting one or both hands, is caused by the impingement, or pinching, of the nerves in the arm, particularly at the wrist. The symptoms can vary from mild hand weakness to pain so severe it can interrupt restful sleep. It commonly affects those people who perform the same motions innumerable times (repetitive stress disorder). However, during pregnancy, CTS usually occurs owing to swelling of the hands (edema) and/or the secretion of the hormone relaxin, which causes all connective tissues of the body to relax in preparation for childbirth. Unfortunately, this powerful hormone also may cause the band of connective tissue around the wrist to relax as well, compromising the integrity of the wrist—the carpal bones—thereby entrapping the nerves. Those women who avoid CTS during pregnancy still might develop it while nursing if they don't keep their wrists straight as they hold the baby.

A related condition, de Quervain's disease, has similar symptoms but affects only the thumbs.

MASSAGE: By the partner. Use oil or lotion. This massage can be performed while mother is seated or lying down. You want to alleviate the pressure on the nerves while lengthening the muscles and reducing pain.

1. Bend her arm at the elbow and hold the affected hand as if you were shaking her hand. Wrap your other hand around her wrist. With her palm facing down, lightly effleurage toward her elbow three times. The return stroke should be a very light glide with practically no pressure. Turn her palm up and repeat the same stroke three more times. You can gently increase your pressure as you repeat the stroke.

2. Using your thumb, effleurage three times down the middle of her forearm, from wrist to elbow. Repeat on the other side of her forearm. There should be no pressure on the return stroke.

3. Place both your thumbs on her wrist, side by side. Apply transverse friction back and forth three times across her wrist. One thumb crosses the joint in an upward stroke as the other one simultaneously crosses in a downward stroke. Turn her hand over and apply friction to the other side of her wrist.

4. Straighten her arm. Apply the same transverse friction stroke at the fleshy part of her forearm, just below her elbow, going across the muscle. This might be a sensitive area, so don't massage too deeply.

5. Bend her arm again and repeat the first effleurage on both sides of her forearm three more times. Make sure the direction of the stroke goes from wrist to elbow with no pressure on the return stroke.

NUTRITION: Vitamin B_6, in conjunction with vitamin B complex, helps reduce water retention. Since it is a safe, water-soluble vitamin, you can take twenty-five to fifty milligrams several times throughout the day.

HINT: Some women get relief from symptoms by wearing a wrist brace. The brace helps to stabilize the wrist joint, taking pressure off the nerves. For those who have to, remember to wear it while nursing.

CHARLEY HORSE—LEG CRAMPS

Charley horses, or cramps of the calf muscles, can be incredibly painful and usually come without warning during sleep or during the morning's first stretch. Since it causes your foot to lock in a pointed manner, flexing it in the opposite direction often alleviates the spasm.

MASSAGE: This can be self-administered, or performed by your partner. Place your finger directly into the middle of the muscle—also called the "belly" of the muscle. Pressing the nodule you feel releases the cramp (see illustration 2.22). Then gently rub up and down the back of the leg. Take care not to work too aggressively, since a deep or vigorous massage after a strong cramp can bring it back. Roll the muscle back and forth, as if you were shaking it (see illustration 2.23). This relaxes the deeper muscle fibers. Circle your foot in both directions and stretch your heel.

If you find that you experience this problem repeatedly, special attention to general leg massage (see the chapter on full body massage) will help keep the muscles toned and flexible. Follow the same basic procedure for toe or thigh cramps.

NUTRITION: A calcium deficiency can be the reason for cramping. Be sure you are eating enough calcium-rich foods. See the section on allergies and sinus congestion for a list of calcium sources. Calcium is vital to the contractile ability of muscles, and a deficiency during pregnancy is not uncommon due to the strain on your body and the developing baby's need for the mineral.

EXERCISE: Any exercise that gently stretches your calf muscles is beneficial.

1. Stand about two feet away from a wall, your feet shoulder width apart. Lean into the wall, keeping the legs straight and heels on the floor (see illustration 2.24). Repeat the stretch a few times.

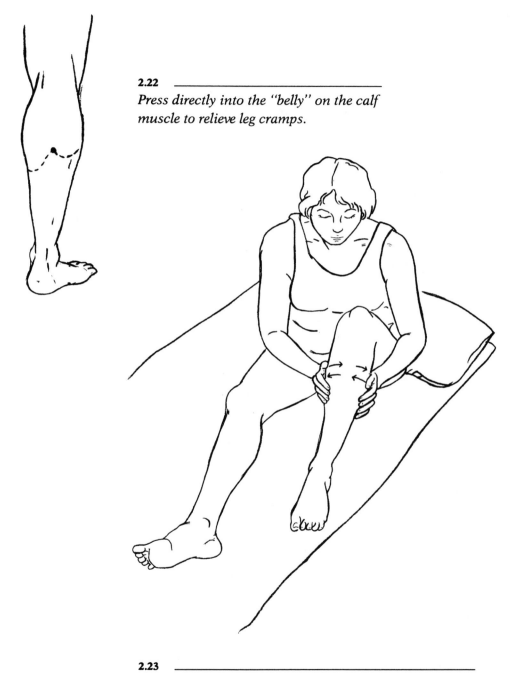

2.22

*Press directly into the "belly" on the calf
muscle to relieve leg cramps.*

2.23

Roll the calf muscle back and forth to ease leg cramps.

2. Sit on the floor and bend one leg for support. Stretch the other leg out in front of you. Inhale. On the exhalation, reach for your toes. Gently pull your toes toward you, keeping your knee straight (see illustration 2.25). You will feel a pull on the hamstring muscles on the back of the thigh. Hold the stretch for ten seconds, breathing normally. Repeat on the other leg.

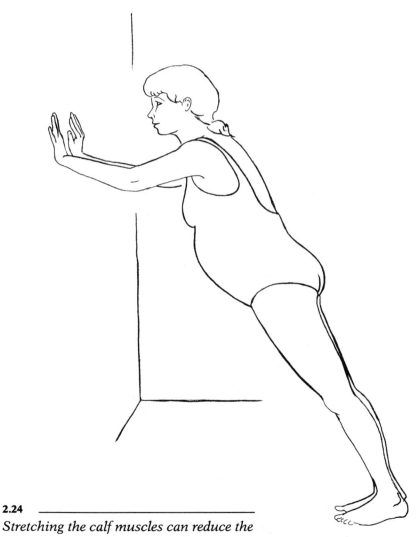

2.24

Stretching the calf muscles can reduce the frequency and severity of leg cramps.

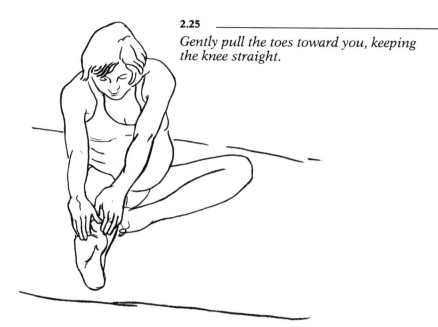

2.25

Gently pull the toes toward you, keeping the knee straight.

CONSTIPATION AND HEARTBURN

Constipation and intestinal gas are common problems of pregnancy. The high levels of progesterone during pregnancy cause relaxation of smooth muscles and reduced intestinal motility (movement also called peristalsis). The pressure of the developing baby on the intestines and certain dietary supplements, especially iron, contribute to this uncomfortable condition. Intestinal gas builds up as the waste products remain in the intestines without being eliminated. There are natural ways to help solve this problem without resorting to commercial laxatives.

Natural papaya juice with digestive enzymes or yogurt with live lactobacillus cultures are easy remedies for this problem. Eating small but frequent meals and drinking at least eight glasses of water daily help rid the body of its waste. Yoga, and stretching and mild aerobics such as walking help to stimulate the peristaltic activity of the intestines. Laxative foods such as fruits, vegetables, whole grains, and bran should also be a daily part of a nutritional dietary regime. Start your day with the juice of half a lemon in a cup of hot water. Honey may be added.

REFLEXOLOGY: Deep abdominal massage cannot be performed during pregnancy, but reflex massage on the feet can be done. The points for the intestines are on both feet. The right foot reflexes the ascending and part of the transverse colon, and the left foot reflexes the transverse and descending colon (see illustration 2.26). Outline the intestines by pressing on the reflex points on the right foot first.

EXERCISES: Daily exercises will relieve constipation. Walking is excellent for general tone and to stimulate peristalsis.

The knee-to-chest position (see illustration 2.27) helps eliminate gas:

• Rest your head and chest on a pillow on the floor, hands under your head. Turn your head to one side.

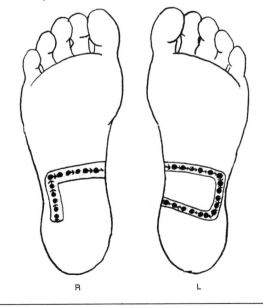

R   L

2.26

Intestinal reflex points to eliminate constipation and heartburn.

- Move your knees as close to your chest as possible. Your backside will be up in the air. Breathe normally. Stay like this for two minutes, and then turn your head in the other direction for another two minutes.

Refer to the section on abdominal pressure. All of these exercises also help relieve gas and constipation.

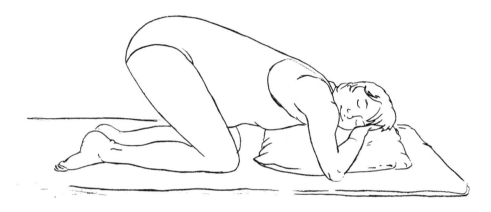

2.27

Knee-to-chest position to eliminate intestinal gas.

HERBS: For heartburn, two to three drops of peppermint oil, rose oil, or sandalwood oil on the tongue are very helpful.

Refer to the section on anemia for iron-rich foods. If the cause of the constipation is the iron supplement you are taking, food sources are suggested to help augment your iron intake.

EDEMA

Edema, or swelling of the extremities, is a common complaint during the last weeks of pregnancy. In the feet, edema is usually a result of fetal head pressure on the pelvic veins, which restricts blood flow from the legs. It is also caused by the extra weight you must support. Although it can be an uncomfortable and sensitive condition, women with edema tend to have slightly larger and fewer premature babies than those who do not develop the condition. For the most part, the swelling is only fluid retention. However, edema can be a symptom of a more serious disorder called toxemia, so your doctor or midwife should be advised of the condition.

Massage's ability to reduce edema is widely accepted. Studies indicate that lymphatic drainage massage increases the reabsorption of edematous fluids and urinary volume.

The posture which provides the most efficient venous blood return is lying on the left side. Elevating the hands and feet above heart level also reduces much of the swelling. Repeat this position several times a day for rest periods of at least fifteen minutes.

MASSAGE: By the partner. Since the uterus presses on the large abdominal vein (vena cava) when the mother is on her back, this treatment offers the best results when she is either lying on her side or sitting upright in a chair or sofa with her legs elevated. The latter is an easier position in which to administer the treatment and offers a more effective massage.

1. This massage is for leg edema. Place a towel under the legs to protect the furniture. Using oil, start with a light stroke and effleurage the thigh from the knee to the hip several times (see illustration 2.28). Repeat the same movement on the back of the leg. Repeat the same stroke, working deeper into the muscles.

2. Using your open palms, make wide circles in opposing directions from the knee to the hip. Work under the thigh, and stroke in the same manner and direction.

3. With your thumbs, make small, alternate circles from the knee to the hip (see illustration 2.29).

4. Effleurage from the ankle to the hip, avoiding direct pressure on the knee. Effleurage from the back of the calf up to the hip. Gradually work deeper.

5. For the foot, lift the leg a few inches and cup your left hand under her heel (see illustration 2.30). Slide your right hand

2.28

Effleurage to reduce leg edema (swelling).

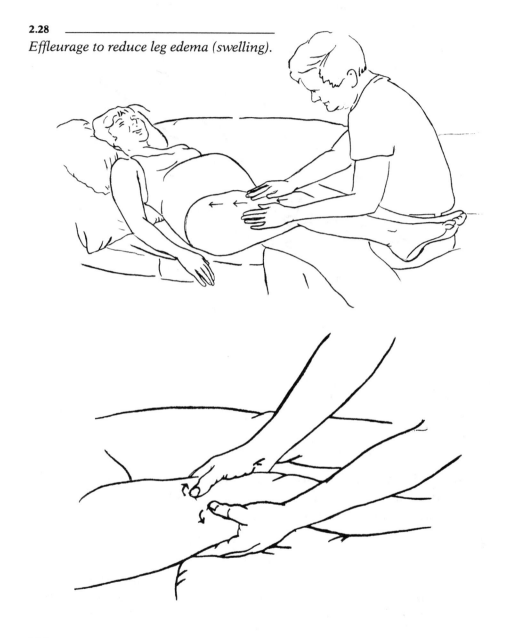

2.29

Alternate thumb circles on the thigh.

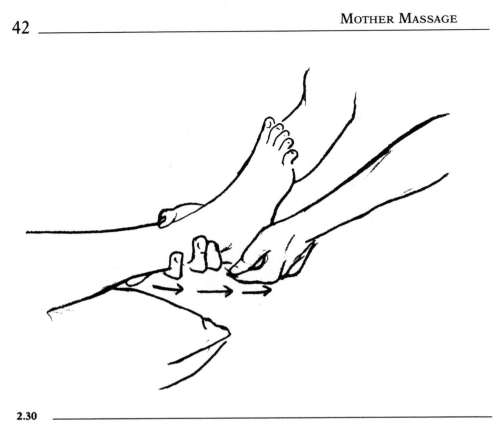

2.30

Alternate hand slide of the Achilles tendon.

along the Achilles tendon toward you. Alternate with the left hand in a flowing motion. Repeat several times. The ankle should be loose and flexible.

6. Put the leg down, to the original position. Place both thumbs on the top of the foot, below the toes, and with your index fingers on the sole of the foot. Since the feet and ankles are probably the most edematous, take special care to begin the treatment lightly. Stroke downward with the pressure on your thumbs at the top of the foot. On the upstroke, the pressure is on the sole of the foot (see illustration 2.31). Repeat in a fluid, gliding manner, getting progressively deeper. Be sure to end with the downstroke.

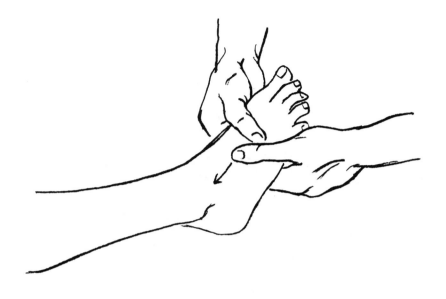

Stroke downward with pressure on the top of the foot. On the upstroke, pressure is on the sole of the foot.

7. Slide down each toe. Rotate each toe three times in both directions.

8. Place one hand under the heel, the other hand grasping her foot below the toes, and rotate the foot three times in each direction (see illustration 2.32).

9. Complete the leg massage with a few more strokes from the ankle to the hip, front and back.

Let her rest with her legs (or arms) elevated. The swelling should be appreciably reduced. Wiggling the toes (or fingers) and ankles (or wrists) also stimulates absorption of the fluid.

The massage treatment to reduce swelling of the arm/hand is based on the same principle as the leg/foot massage—that is, to

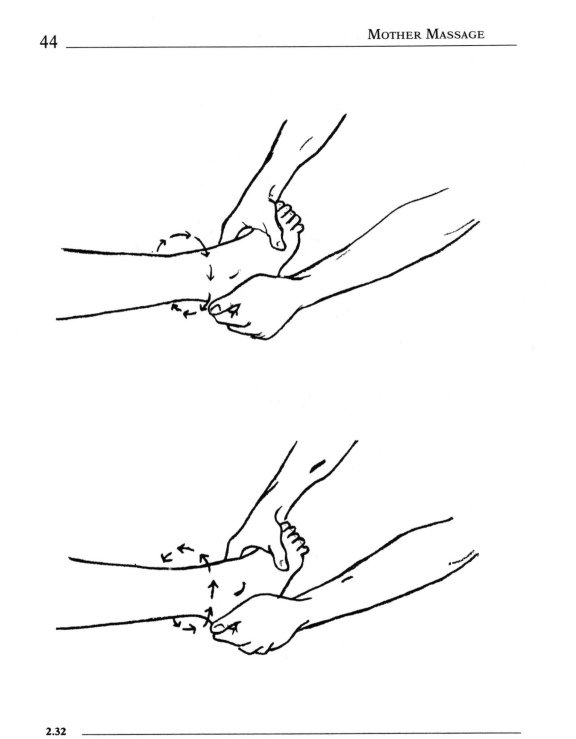

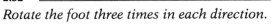

2.32

Rotate the foot three times in each direction.

facilitate drainage of the excess fluid, you begin the massage at the part of the limb closest to the trunk (the proximal end) and work farther down the limb to the portion of the extremity farthest from the trunk (the distal end). The direction of the stroke is always toward the trunk.

The arm massage can be done seated or side-lying following the same sequence and strokes as the leg massage, substituting upper arm for thigh and forearm for calf. Make sure you massage all around the limb, just as you did for the leg.

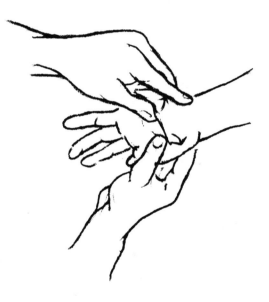

2.33

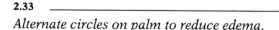

Alternate circles on palm to reduce edema.

The hand massage is only slightly different from the foot massage.

1. Using your thumb, massage the space between each bone on the top of the hand.

2. Slide down each finger, and rotate each finger three times in both directions.

3. Turn the hand over, palm facing up. Make small, alternate circles on the mother's palm (see illustration 2.33). Support her hand underneath with your fingers.

4. Turn her hand over again and gently press each finger back, stretching it carefully.

5. Complete the arm massage with a few more strokes from the wrist to the shoulder, front and back (see illustration 2.34).

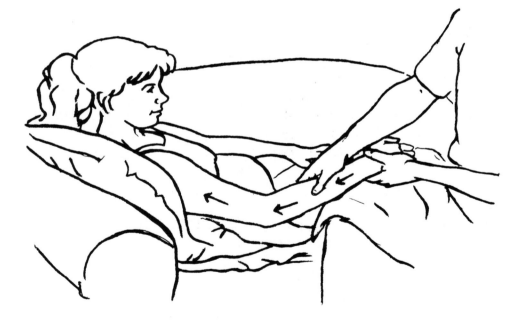

2.34
Effleurage of the arm.

NUTRITION: Although progesterone secreted during pregnancy increases the sodium excreted by the kidneys, excessive salt and sodium should be avoided. Follow a nutritious, balanced diet, including salt in moderation.

Drink at least eight glasses of water daily.

Vitamin B_6, in conjunction with vitamin B complex, is helpful to reduce water retention; twenty-five to fifty milligrams daily are all you need.

HINT: Soaking your hands and feet is relaxing and soothing and reduces the swelling. Add half a cup of Epsom salts to two cups of boiling water. Let the salt dissolve, and then add it to the warm water in your basin. The water level should be up to your ankles. If you want to bathe in the salts, add two cups of salts to four cups of boiling water to your bathwater.

FATIGUE

Pregnancy slows down your metabolism, so you feel tired. Listen to your body, and rest as often as possible. Hormonal changes are contributing factors to fatigue, as is the extra weight you are carrying. Increased blood volume, which slows down circulation; shortness of breath; constipation; anemia; and nutritional deficiencies all play a part in making you feel languid, listless, and tired.

MASSAGE: By the partner. A light, full body massage (as described in the chapter on full body massage) will combat fatigue. Since massage improves circulation, more oxygen is absorbed into the tissues of the body. Waste products are more readily eliminated, and muscle stress is reduced. The afterglow of total relaxation is especially rejuvenating. Massage will also induce sleep, the very medicine your body craves.

EXERCISE: Any exercise that improves overall circulation (without further exhausting you) is beneficial. Make sure that your doctor or midwife is aware of any exercise program in which you partake. If you have always been active, continue doing so. An abrupt change in your activity can actually contribute to your fatigue. When your body is used to producing the endorphins (which give you the "runner's high") from regular exercise, sudden cessation of exercise causes a depression in the secretion of this hormone. That in turn can translate into fatigue.

If you have never exercised before, this is a good time to start. Check with your doctor or midwife and then seek out a class that specializes in exercise for pregnant women.

N U T R I T I O N : Proper nutrition will keep your energy level high. Iron is an important nutrient during pregnancy. (See the section on anemia for a list of iron-rich foods.) Iron prevents anemia, which often causes fatigue. Protein, another essential element to ward off tiredness, is found in meat, fish, poultry, eggs, cheese, and legumes. To be sure you have enough protein for yourself and your developing baby, have a serving of this food group during meals and at snack time.

HEADACHES

Hormonal changes may cause headaches as well as sinus congestion, constipation, and emotional stress.

M A S S A G E : By the partner. Have the mother lie down, and prop pillows under her knees and head. Make sure the light is dim and the room is quiet. Let her rest calmly for a few minutes with a cold compress on her forehead.

The section on allergies and sinus congestion demonstrates how to alleviate a sinus headache. Many of the same techniques are applicable to general (or migraine) headache relief.

1. Sit at your partner's head. Remove the compress, and gently cradle her head in your hands, under her neck. On her exhalation, lift her head gently a few inches off the pillow and pull easily on her neck, giving a slight traction (see illustration

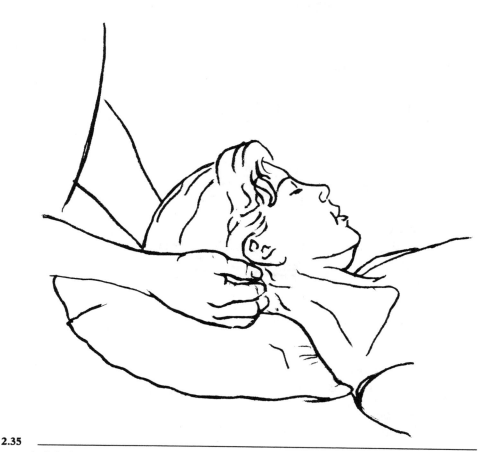

2.35

Gently lift the expectant mother's head off the pillow and pull with slight traction.

2.35). Hold this position for several breaths as she relaxes into this position.

2. Softly put her head back on the pillow. Using your fingertips and thumbs, "shampoo" her scalp. This will increase circulation to her head and reduce muscle tension.

3. With both thumbs, press down in half-inch increments on the center part of her scalp. Work with her breath, pressing down with each exhalation. Start from the hairline and work to the crown of the head. If any point is particularly sensitive, stay on that point for several breaths.

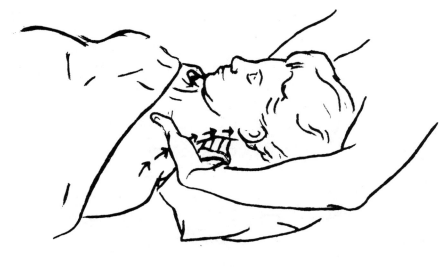

Effleurage from the shoulders to the back of the neck.

4. Effleurage from her shoulders to the back of her neck (see illustration 2.36). Repeat this several more times.

5. Squeeze the muscles at the back of her neck. Repeat the effleurage to her neck.

HERBS: Nettle tea, three tablespoons to one cup, or yerba santa tea, one teaspoon to one cup, are both very effective for combating headaches.

HEMORRHOIDS

Hemorrhoids are varicose veins of the anus. The pressure of the developing baby can cause hemorrhoids to swell, itch, and burn. Straining during a bowel movement is also a contributing factor. In addition, pushing during labor promotes hemorrhoids to develop.

Although there is no specific massage for the treatment of hemorrhoids, a general massage will promote better circulation and thereby help reduce the swelling.

REFLEXOLOGY: By the partner. The reflex point on the feet for the treatment of hemorrhoids is on the heel (see illustration 2.37). Press the point on both feet for fifteen to thirty seconds repeatedly. Treat each foot for five minutes. Refer to the colon reflex points on page 38, as they will stimulate an easier bowel movement.

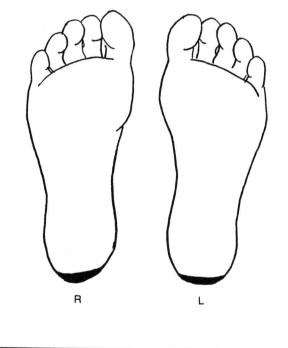

R   L

2.37

The reflex point for hemorrhoids is on the heels of both feet.

EXERCISES: The same Kegel exercises you will do for vaginal control help pump the blood out of the engorged pelvic veins. The idea of these exercises is primarily to develop control of the sphincter muscles in the groin to facilitate recovery after labor. To do these exercises, tighten the vaginal and anal muscles. If you find them difficult to locate, sit on the toilet and release a small amount of urine. Stop "midstream." Release again. These are the sphincter muscles of the vagina. The anus will also contract during this process.

S H I A T S U P O I N T : At the crown of the head you will locate the point for hemorrhoids (see illustration 2.38). Press three times for fifteen seconds each.

H I N T : Witch hazel, lemon juice, or vitamin E applied directly to the hemorrhoids will help shrink them. Vitamin B_6 deficiency seems to contribute to development of hemorrhoids. Make sure that your diet includes a minimum of ten milligrams of vitamin B_6 along with vitamin B complex.

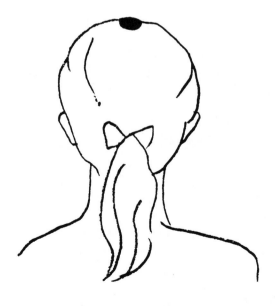

2.38

Shiatsu point for treatment of hemorrhoids.

INSOMNIA

Insomnia during pregnancy is due to a myriad of reasons—physical, dietary, emotional, psychological, etc. But the bottom line is that you need your rest.

MASSAGE: By the partner. A general, full body massage, or relief from any of the specific problems that might be interrupting sleep is excellent in reducing stress and promoting deep relaxation.

NUTRITION: Make sure your diet has sufficient calcium. A cup of hot milk with honey is calming and promotes sleep.

HERBS: One cup of hops or scullcap tea (found in health food stores) will relax you and induce sleep. Many women find a cup of chamomile tea very soothing before bed.

MORNING SICKNESS AND NAUSEA

When you read the section on contraindications of massage, you learned that massage is not indicated when morning sickness or nausea is present. However, you can make certain dietary adjustments to minimize the effects of morning sickness.

For example, drinking red raspberry leaf tea (found in health food stores) is very helpful and rather tasty. Peppermint tea also is an effective treatment. Drink often throughout the day.

Nausea is sometimes due to an empty stomach, so small, frequent meals should be *de rigueur*. Protein snacks at bedtime seem to help because protein digests slowly enough that there is always something in the stomach until morning. Keeping rice cakes or crackers by the bed also seems to reduce morning sickness.

However, until your hormones normalize, usually by the second trimester you will have to combat the nausea in the best way possible. These suggestions seem to help many women.

Some women get relief from these symptoms by pressing on the acupuncture point, Pericardium 6, found on both forearms. To locate this point, measure 1½ inches below the crease of your wrists, in the middle of your forearms. Press six to ten seconds, repeating six to ten times. Wristbands sold in most pharmacies to prevent motion sickness can be worn to reduce the nausea without unwanted side effects. A small plastic button in the wristband stimulates this point.

SCIATICA

Sciatica is a painful inflammation of the sciatic nerve. During pregnancy it occurs due to the pressure or position of the growing baby. The pain courses along the path of the nerve, which is in the middle of the back of the leg. It affects only one leg.

Be sure to advise your physician or health care provider of this condition so that other pathologies or causes may be ruled out. Sciatica caused by pregnancy disappears after birthing. However, massage during pregnancy is very beneficial to reduce the pain.

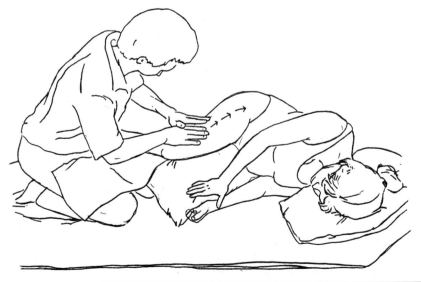

2.39

Effleurage of the leg.

Since lying on her back might exacerbate the pain, the mother should be lying on the unaffected side for this treatment, pillows placed between her knees and under her head. Massage only the affected leg.

MASSAGE: By the partner. Do each stroke three times. Use massage oil.

1. Effleurage the entire leg front and back, including the gluteal (buttocks) region (see illustration 2.39).

2. Circular kneading with one hand, including the gluteal region, relaxes the inflammation. Place your other hand on the mother's hip, avoiding any deep pressure.

3. Using your thumbs, make small circles, tracing along her sacrum (the triangular bone at the base of the spine).

4. With both thumbs, one above the other, make small, transverse strokes (friction) down the middle of the back of the leg, along the path of the nerve (see illustration 2.40). This stroke is especially important to reduce the inflammation.

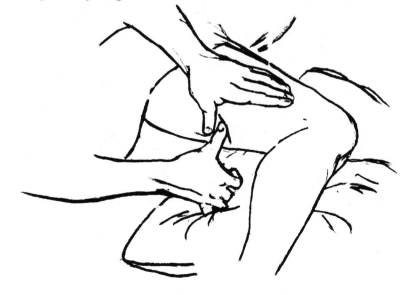

2.40

Transverse friction on the back of the thigh to reduce sciatic pain.

5. Repeat the first stroke of effleurage up the back of the leg.

6. Tap gently with the back of your hand all along the back of the leg. The gluteals are next. Concentrate on the topmost portion of the back of her thigh, directly under the gluteals (see illustration 2.41).

7. Finish the massage with a gentle nerve stroke, from the buttocks to the foot (see illustration 2.42).

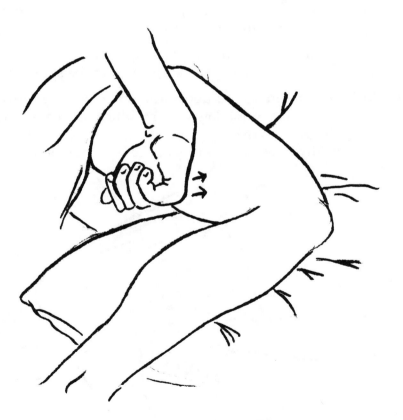

2.41

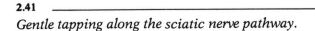

Gentle tapping along the sciatic nerve pathway.

2.42

Nerve stroke for the treatment of sciatica.

REFLEXOLOGY: Hold each point for fifteen seconds. Release for five seconds. Repeat three times. The mother can be seated in a chair for this.

1. Press the area around the outside of the anklebone very carefully (see illustration 2.43a).

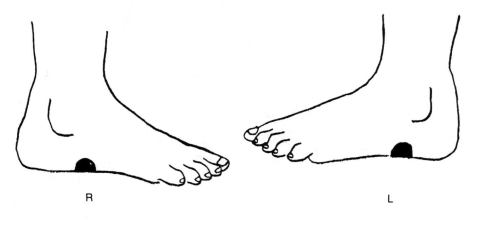

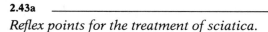

2.43a

Reflex points for the treatment of sciatica.

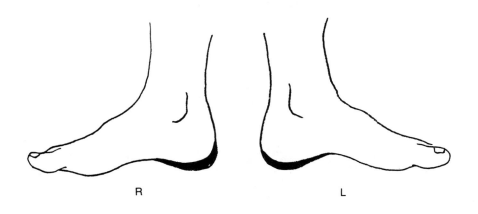

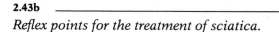

2.43b

Reflex points for the treatment of sciatica.

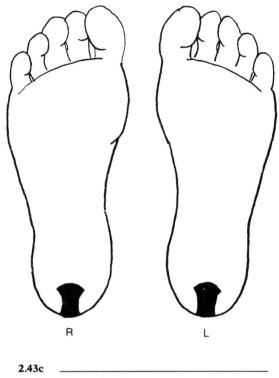

2.43c

Reflex points for the treatment of sciatica.

2. The hip reflexes around the heel play an important role in controlling sciatic pain. Press gently on the back of the heel (see illustration 2.43b).

3. Press the center of the back of the heel (see illustration 2.43c).

SORE NIPPLES

Preparing your body for nursing by toughening your nipples is one way to avoid soreness. (See the section on breast soreness for more details.) However, it is impossible to ascertain how demanding a feeder your baby will be, and sometimes sore nipples result.

HERBS: Two drops of rose oil in one ounce of sweet almond oil applied to the nipple will ease the tenderness. Be sure to clean yourself before nursing.

STRETCH MARKS

There is nothing concrete to determine who will develop stretch marks during pregnancy. Studies indicate that whenever there is a disturbance in the endocrine system, either due to pregnancy or rapid weight gain and/or loss, the integrity of the skin becomes lax. Once this happens, the stretch marks will not disappear. They will, however, fade in time.

HERBS: A topical massage with vitamin E, coconut oil, or olive oil may hasten the healing. A massage oil made up of twenty-five drops of lavender oil with an optional five drops of neroli oil in two ounces of wheat germ oil (to be used after the first trimester) may also promote faster healing and fading of the marks.

VARICOSE VEINS

During pregnancy, the blood vessels (veins and arteries) are less resilient due to the increase of progesterone. They become lax, and the pressure on the pelvic veins compounded with impeded venous return from the legs cause the veins to bulge.

Massage is *never* given directly on top of the varicose veins, but a general leg massage will help reduce the engorgement of the veins. Follow the same treatment for edema, taking special care to avoid direct pressure on the weakened veins.

EXERCISE: Walking or any form of nonstress activity is excellent therapy.

Elevation of the limb helps take the pressure off the veins.

NUTRITION: Include vitamin C (100 milligrams) and vitamin E (600 I.U.) in your daily supplementation to help reduce varicosities.

CHAPTER 3

FULL BODY MASSAGE

*T*he experience of pregnancy should not be solely defined on the basis of the discomforts the expectant mother may encounter. The full body massage that follows allows the mother and her partner to enjoy a very sensuous, loving, and tender way to maintain optimum health and energy levels. This massage offers couples a unique and pleasurable opportunity to intensify their emotional involvement with each other and can serve as foreplay to lovemaking.

For the expectant mother, who may develop a poor self-image as her body grows, massage provides an unparalleled way of receiving acceptance for her ever-changing body. When lovemaking is uncomfortable or undesired, massage can provide an intimate substitute.

For the expectant father, whose emotional stress and sympathetic physical changes are often overlooked, this massage provides a special time to affirm and accept his feelings and reduce his anxieties. Although the treatment is designed to follow the precepts of pregnancy massage and will often repeat the procedures found in Chapter 2, the father will still benefit from the care and attention.

Along with the emotional support massage provides, many physical benefits accompany any treatment. As you experienced from the massage techniques in Chapter 2, many of the discomforts of pregnancy can be reduced and often eliminated with massage. In addition, massage will:

- relax muscle spasms and relieve tension

- dilate blood vessels, thereby improving circulation and enhancing lymphatic drainage

- reabsorb waste products caused by strenuous activity or injury

- improve muscle tone

- promote deeper relaxation because of its sedative effect on the nervous system

- stretch connective tissue (ligaments and tendons)

- improve circulation and nutrition to the joints, making them more flexible and less prone to injury

Communication through touch is very powerful. A lot can be said from the touch of a hand. If you think you haven't yet developed the stamina to massage your partner's entire body, start with the most tense area. It is very often the back and the neck. The more you practice, the stronger you will get, and the more endurance you will develop.

For fairness sake, the techniques have been described as if the father were the recipient of the massage. Specific accommodations for the mother are listed where applicable.

It is important for the provider to maintain a comfortable posture during all the techniques. An extra pillow under the knees can provide additional support on a hard floor.

BACK MASSAGE

The back massage technique for the mother in the later stages of pregnancy appears in Chapter 2. If she can still lie on her stomach, she can receive the same treatment listed below.

Have your partner lie face down on a comfortable surface with arms at his sides. Prop a pillow under his ankles. Kneel at his side. Warm the oil between your hands.

1. Effleurage from the base of his spine up and around both shoulders (see illustration 3.1). Repeat this stroke several times with increased pressure.

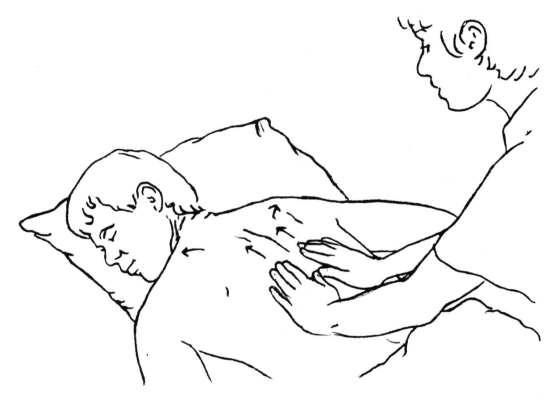

3.1

Effleurage of the back.

2. Circle all around his shoulders, increasing the pressure. Stroke up and down his neck.

3. Gently squeeze the muscles on the top of the shoulder.

4. With your thumbs, make small, alternate circles (petrissage) along the border of the shoulder blades (see illustration 3.2). With an open hand, make larger circles all around the shoulder, as you did before.

5. Make alternate thumb circles on his sacrum, the triangular bone at the base of his spine (see illustration 3.3).

6. Finish his back massage with several of the same gliding effleurage strokes you began with, and complete the back massage with a gentle nerve stroke, from shoulders to hips.

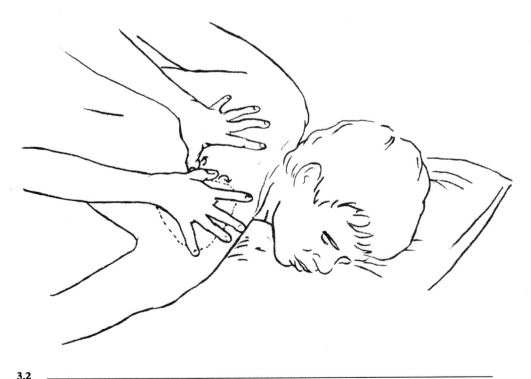

3.2 _____

Alternate thumb circles along the shoulder blades.

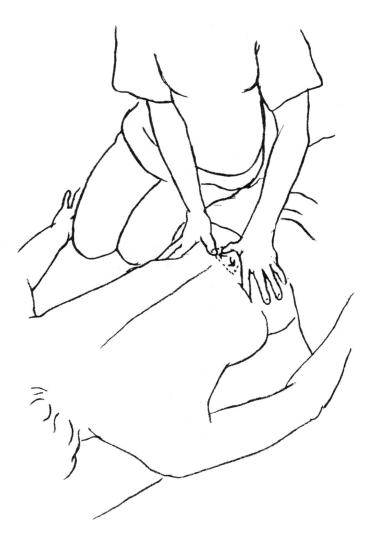

3.3

Alternate thumb circles on the sacrum.

BACK OF LEGS

As long as the father is prone, you might as well proceed to the back of his legs. Move down to knee level.

1. Lightly apply the oil with a long, gliding effleurage from his ankle to his buttocks. Repeat the stroke, getting deeper each time. Avoid direct pressure to the back of his knee.

2. Using your open palms, make wide circles in opposing directions, from knee to hip. With your outside hand, circle the outside of his buttock. With your thumbs, make small, alternate circles in the middle of his thigh, from knee to hip (see illustration 3.4).

3. Using open palms, make wide circles in opposing directions on his calf, all the way up his thigh. With your thumbs, make small, alternate circles in the middle of his calf, all the way up his thigh.

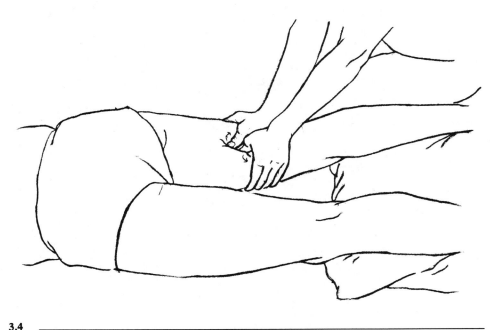

3.4 _____

Alternate circles on the back of the thigh.

4. Move down to his foot. Hold the ankle with one hand and alternately glide toward you (see illustration 3.5). Secure the foot and place your thumbs next to each other on his heel. Glide down his foot five times, starting at his heel and ending at each toe.

5. Repeat the first effleurage, from ankle to buttocks, a few more times. End with a gentle nerve stroke, gliding down from his hip to his foot. Repeat the same sequence on the other leg.

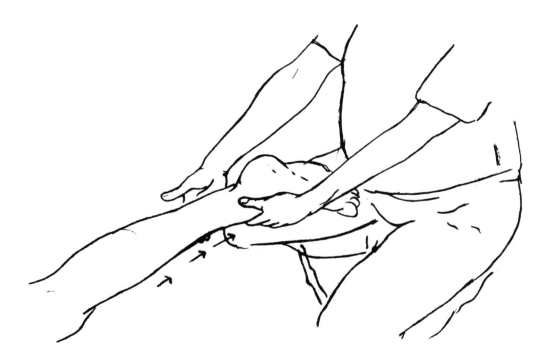

3.5

Alternate glide of the foot.

HEAD AND FACE

The father should turn over. Place a pillow under his knees, and keep a pillow in reserve for his head when the neck massage is over. The mother can also lie on her back, as long as she is comfortable.

The provider should position herself seated comfortably at the father's head.

HEAD

1. "Shampoo" his scalp with your fingertips.

2. With your thumbs, apply pressure down the center of his head, from hairline to crown.

FACE

1. Gently glide from his chin to his jaw. If he has a beard, you can press his jaw with your fingers.

2. Make small circles with your fingertips at his jaw.

3. Glide your fingertips under his cheekbones, from nose to temples.

4. Make small circles at his temples.

5. Using your thumbs, outline his eyebrows. Move above his eyebrows and stretch his forehead with the same stroke. Continue moving upward toward his hairline, stretching out to his temples.

NECK

1. Cup both hands under his neck and gently stretch his head. Hold for three seconds and gently release.

2. Place both hands on his chest, fingertips together. Stroke across his chest, over his shoulders, and up his neck (see illustration 3.6). Repeat this stroke several times, getting progressively deeper.

3. Turn his head to one side and stroke down the side of his neck several times. Repeat on the other side.

4. Stroke under his neck, one hand following the other. Place the pillow under his head when the neck massage is completed.

3.6

Stroke across the chest, over the shoulders, and up the neck.

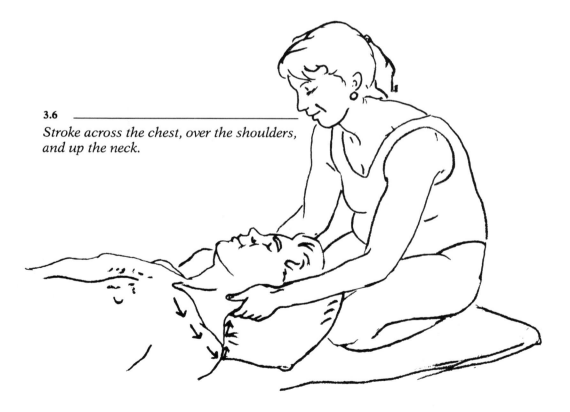

CHEST

If the mother's breasts are sore, or if she is lactating, it is advisable to ask about the tenderness before proceeding with the massage. And if the father has a hairy chest, this massage may be difficult for the provider or uncomfortable if his hair is pulled. Use extra lubrication to avoid this problem.

1. With the heels of your palms, stroke alternately from shoulder to breastbone (see illustration 3.7).

2. With your thumbs, alternately stroke from one side of his chest across to the other shoulder.

3. Repeat the first stroke three more times.

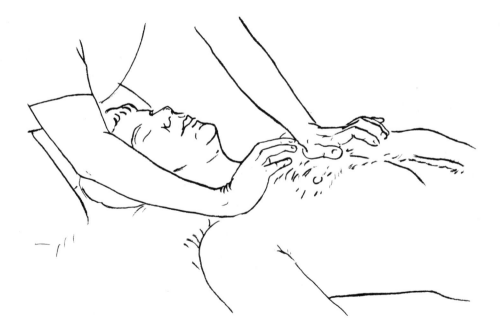

3.7 _____
Alternate palm stroke of the chest.

ABDOMEN

Caution is advised when massaging a pregnant woman's abdomen. A light touch is very relaxing and soothing and can indeed be felt by the baby. This is also a unique opportunity for the expectant father to communicate with the child in utero. Many fathers talk to their babies when massaging the abdomen. The baby can hear.

Position yourself at the father's side. Make sure that all strokes are in a clockwise direction.

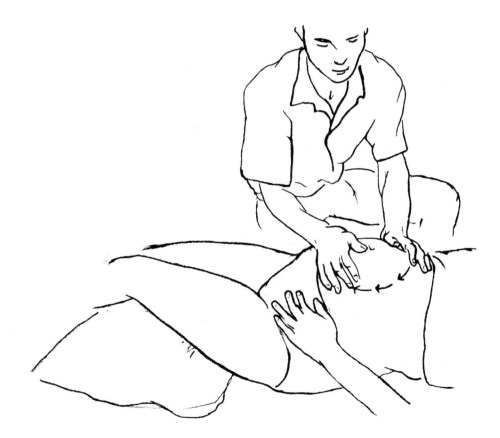

3.8a

Abdominal effleurage. Always follow a clockwise direction.

1. Place one hand beneath his ribs, the other beneath his navel. Circle around the abdomen with both hands (see illustration 3.8a). When they cross, pick up one hand and place it opposite the other (see illustration 3.8b). Continue the stroke in a clockwise direction.

2. Place your flat palms on his ribs and glide outward.

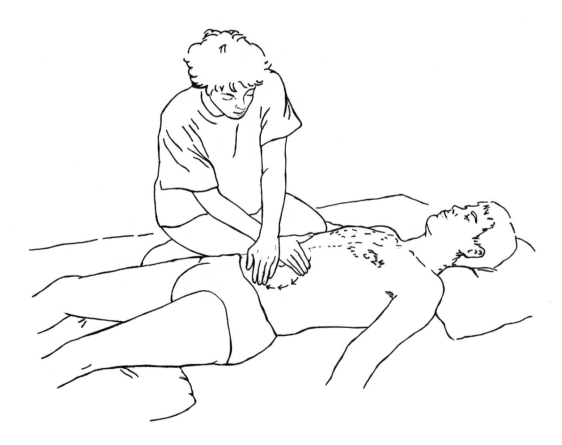

3.8b _____

Abdominal effleurage. Always follow a clockwise direction.

ARMS

1. Apply the oil by gliding from his wrist to his shoulder. You might find it easier to hold his wrist to secure the arm in place. Turn his arm over and effleurage the inside of the arm.

2. Effleurage from elbow to shoulder. Glide up the top of the shoulder to his neck (see illustration 3.9).

3. Effleurage from wrist to shoulder.

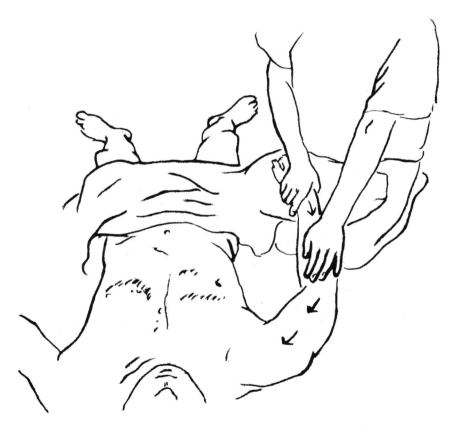

3.9

Arm effleurage.

4. With alternate thumb circles, petrissage from his wrist to his shoulder (see illustration 3.10).

5. Lift his wrist and massage the palm of his hand with alternate thumb circles. Glide down each finger.

6. Replace his arm and repeat the first effleurage, from wrist to shoulder.

7. Apply a gentle nerve stroke from his shoulder to fingers, signaling the end of the arm massage.

Before changing sides, massage the front of his leg.

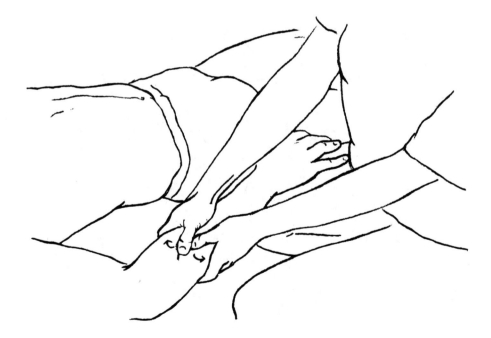

3.10 _____

Alternate thumb circles on the arm.

FRONT OF LEGS

Move down to knee level.

1. Apply the oil with an effleurage from ankle to hip. Avoid direct pressure on the knee. Repeat the stroke, getting progressively deeper (see illustration 3.11).

2. Using open palms, make wide circles in opposing directions from knee to hip.

3. With your thumbs, make small, alternate circles from knee to hip.

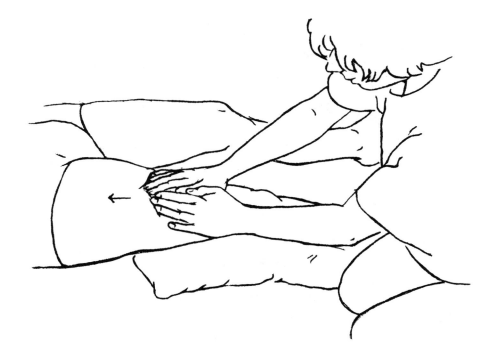

3.11

Effleurage of the leg. Avoid direct pressure on the knee.

4. Effleurage from ankle to hip. Make small circles with your fingertips on the inside and outside of his calf (see illustration 3.12).

5. Circle the knee with your fingertips.

6. Effleurage the entire leg.

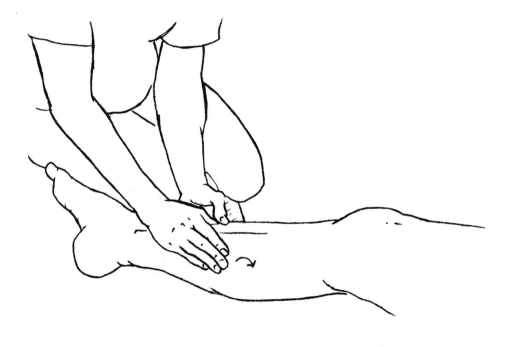

3.12
Circular kneading of the sides of the leg.

7. Move down to the foot. Gently lift the leg a few inches off the floor and cup your left hand under his heel. Slide your right hand along the Achilles tendon, pulling toward you. Alternate with the left hand in a flowing motion (see illustration 3.13).

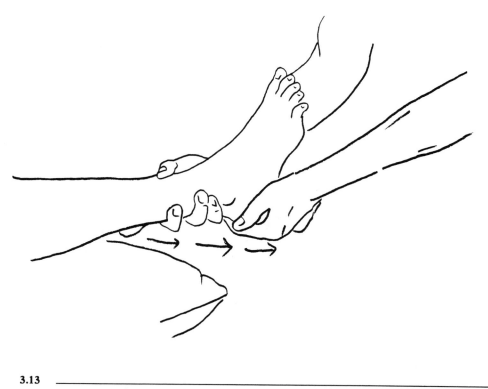

3.13

Alternate hand slide of the Achilles tendon.

8. Put the leg down. Place both thumbs on the top of the foot, below the toes, with your index finger on the sole of the foot. Stroke downward, with pressure on your thumbs. On the upstroke, the pressure is on the sole of the foot.

9. Slide down each toe.

10. Repeat the full leg effleurage. Complete the leg massage with a nerve stroke from hip to foot.

Move to the other side and finish the full body massage with the other arm and leg. If the father isn't blissed out by now, he's beyond redemption!

CHAPTER 4

GETTING READY FOR BIRTHING

*I*n the final few weeks before birthing, perineal massage techniques and Kegel exercises are performed by the expectant mother to make birthing as unstrained and easy as possible.

The perineum, the area between the vagina and anus, stretches as the baby is born. (Your doctor might see fit to perform an episiotomy, which is an incision to enlarge the vaginal opening and to prevent perineal tearing. If this is the case, a local anesthesia will be given. The stitches to repair the incision are absorbed within fifteen to twenty days.)

PERINEAL MASSAGE: The purpose of perineal massage is increased relaxation and elasticity of the pelvic floor and improved chances of intact perineal delivery, lessening the chances of an episiotomy. It helps to promote rapid healing and tissue recovery after birthing. The massage also teaches the mother how to identify the muscles that should relax during delivery. The massage will increase blood and lymphatic flow, stretch the perineal muscle fibers, and increase elasticity. It will nourish the perineum and optimize tissue integrity.

Tribal women understood the need to stretch the perineum prior to delivery and employed varied techniques to achieve this purpose. In some cases, steaming or bathing this sensitive area preceded labor; shallow baths of herbs were common among some tribes weeks before delivery; women in other tribes squatted over herbal steam baths to relax the perineum. In many cases, lubrications of many varieties, including animal fat, sap, and fruits were applied directly to the perineum to prevent tearing.

The perineal massage is usually self-administered, although it can be done by the birthing partner. The massage should be done in a slow, rhythmical manner.

There are some contraindications to perineal massage:

1. If there are pelvic varicose veins.

2. If there are active herpes lesions.

3. Make sure to avoid the urinary tract opening.

Do the massage daily for at least five minutes, starting in your week thirty four (approximately six weeks prior to birthing). Use a warmed oil rich in vitamin E, such as wheat germ oil, or break a vitamin E capsule into vegetable oil. Get into a comfortable position, seated against pillows for support. Make sure your hands are thoroughly washed, nails are short, and jewelry is removed. Empty your bladder before beginning.

1. Dip a sterile gauze pad into the warmed oil and place the pad on the perineum to loosen the tissues and make the area more pliable.

2. Dip your index fingers or thumbs into the oil and rub it a bit more vigorously into the perineum.

3. Using your thumbs (or the most comfortable fingers), place them 1 to 1½ inches into your vagina and press downward toward the rectum and out to the sides (see illustration 4.1). Stretch gently and firmly, keeping a steady pressure until you

feel a slight tingling or burning sensation. Hold this for about two minutes, when the area will become a little numb and the tingling will subside.

4. While maintaining steady pressure, move in a rhythmic U-formation, back and forth over the lower half of your vagina (see illustration 4.1). Gently stretch outward as you do this for approximately three to four minutes. This helps stretch the skin as the baby will do during birth, and you will feel a similar burning as the baby's head crowns.

5. Concentrate on relaxing. Breathing helps release the muscles. With daily massage you will notice greater elasticity as your due date approaches.

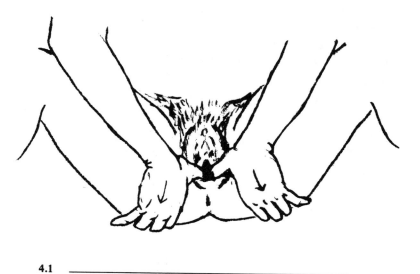

4.1

Massage to stretch perineal tissues prior to birthing.

HEALING PERINEUM SITZ BATH: After the birth, a very effective sitz bath for healing the perineum is: two drops of cypress oil and four drops of lavender oil in a large bowl or shallow bath. Sit for a minimum of fifteen minutes daily for one week to ten days, or until healing is complete.

KEGEL EXERCISES: Before and after birthing, employ Kegel exercises to tone the stretched muscles. These muscle contractions are performed as if you were trying to stop urination. As a matter of fact, one way to practice identifying the muscles involved is to release a small amount of urine and stop. Release some more and stop. These are the muscles that tighten when controlling the flow of urine. You can also practice this tightening action while making love with your partner, which has the added bonus of pleasing both of you.

Doing Kegel exercises will help you relax more efficiently for the perineal stretching of labor because the muscles will be better toned. Dr. Kegel states that perineal muscles demonstrate amazing recuperative powers and that this sphincteric zone is quite elastic and resilient. Exercise is a very important factor in restoring functional capacity to any skeletal muscle; therefore, in postpartum care these exercises are of particular importance.

Once you are familiar with the muscles involved (vaginal opening and anus), practice these exercises for three- to five-minute intervals at least three times a day and more frequently after birthing.

CHAPTER 5

LABOR MASSAGE

SIGNS OF LABOR: Women often wonder if they will know when they are really going into labor. This is not as farfetched as it may seem, since false labor is often misinterpreted by overanxious expectant parents.

During the last months of pregnancy, the uterus contracts in preparation for labor. These Braxton-Hicks contractions (the same ones you experienced at the onset of your pregnancy) are not actual labor, but they tone the uterus and keep it strong for the ensuing labor. These contractions differ from true labor since they have no regularity and rarely get stronger. True labor contractions are regular and get increasingly stronger and closer together. Braxton-Hicks contractions will often stop if you alter your activity, whereas labor contractions get stronger if you walk around. (Being ambulatory can also stimulate labor and help to position the baby. Native Americans of Arizona said that a woman should do as much walking as possible to make her labor easier. If she couldn't walk on her own, she had assistants helping her.)

As labor gets closer, there will be noticeable changes in your body. The baby drops (known as engagement) deeper into the birth canal, which causes the uterus to move down as well. This is called lightening. As a result of this movement, you are carrying lower and the baby's activity lessens, since there isn't as much room to kick and stretch. You will also notice that the shortness of breath has eased and that you suffer from less indigestion. However, you might experience more pressure in the groin and aches in your legs.

Prior to birthing there is an increase in discharge of mucus from the vagina and an increase in fluid from your breasts. Colostrum, which will be the baby's first milklike nourishment, rich in antibodies and nutrients, is the name of this secretion. It is a watery liquid.

The plug of mucus, which filled the opening of the cervix and protected the baby from germs, shows. This means it discharges, releasing blood and mucus. The "waters" that break are the amniotic fluids that surrounded the baby in the uterus.

Some women actually lose a few pounds prior to labor. Others experience a surge of energy and start preparing and cleaning the house for the baby's arrival. This is what is known as the nesting instinct.

In the Amazon region, the expectant mother recognizes large veins on her abdomen as a sign of impending labor. Native Americans of North America knew that birth was a short time off when the mother was sick in the evening and had pains in her lower back.

The three stages of labor are as follows:

FIRST STAGE: The cervix thins out, or effaces, and opens, or dilates. This can also happen prior to labor. The contractions are persistent and can last fourteen to twenty-four hours or longer for first-time mothers (primaparas) and an average of seven hours for women with previous births (multiparas). Being ambulatory helps speed up labor. When the cervix has dilated to 7 cm. the transition period begins. Transition continues until the cervix has dilated to 10 cm., signaling the end of the first stage of labor.

SECOND STAGE: This can last one to three hours. Bearing

down offers relief. You are actively pushing during this stage. The baby is moving into the vagina, and as the head crowns, you will recognize the burning sensation you felt while doing the perineal massage. Your baby is born during the second stage.

THIRD STAGE: Although the baby has been born, the uterus continues to contract to expel the placenta, also called the afterbirth. Nursing stimulates these contractions and can shorten the time for the third stage of labor, which usually takes ten to thirty minutes. Nursing also helps with maternal bonding.

Margaret Mead noted that birthing in Samoa was a group effort. Twenty to thirty people stayed with the laboring woman, helping her with a celebration of humor, games, jokes, and support. In Malaya as well, friends would attend the birth and take turns massaging the mother's belly.

Navajos of Arizona always had a woman attending the birth to support and massage the mother during labor. In addition to easing the labor, massage was almost universally used in tribal societies to reposition malpresentations, or breech births.

In our modern society, where fathers are permitted into the delivery rooms, massage during labor can be employed once again to relieve muscle tension (especially in back labor), offer active physical and emotional support, and make the birthing process as comfortable as possible.

MASSAGE DURING LABOR

Some women prefer not to be touched during labor, but for those who do, labor massage offers relief from muscle contractions, reduction in pain and anxieties, and increase in self-assurance, and will also provide loving encouragement and support. In addition, it can promote a speedier birth.

The Journal of Nurse-Midwifery[1] cited a 1984 study on touch received during labor that said that all the participating women responded positively to the physical contact. The study indicated

1. Vol. 31, No. 6, (November/December 1986, pp. 270–276).

that the most helpful time to touch was during the transition stage of labor, when anxiety is highest, and that the overall opinion was that touch gave the women more confidence and helped them to cope.

The feeling of being supported and comforted by the person touching, the care and reassurance offered by that contact, and the closeness and trust felt toward the caregiver are high on the list of responses to the treatment. There was also an important sense of self-control, because the laboring women were able to meet their physical needs through the contact. Many women spoke of feeling safe because of the care.

HERBS: An aromatic massage oil especially for labor is very relaxing and deeply penetrating: twelve drops of clary sage oil, five drops of rose oil, and five drops of ylang-ylang in two fluid ounces of vegetable oil.

LOWER BACK: To relieve her lower back discomfort, position the mother on her side, with a pillow under her head and between her knees. If she feels more comfortable seated in front of you, the father will have to accommodate this position by working behind her.

1. Using alternate thumb circles, massage her sacrum, the triangular bone at the base of the spine, with as much pressure as she finds comfortable (see illustration 5.1). Continue the movement up each side of her spine, stopping at waist level.

2. Holding on to her shoulder with one hand, effleurage up one side of the spine, circling around her shoulder. Repeat several times on one side before massaging the other side. The mother does not have to turn over if she is side-lying, although access to her other shoulder will be limited.

3. Press, using both thumbs, the points one inch on either side of the spine, starting from the sacrum, moving up in one-inch increments (see illustration 5.2). Hold each point for five seconds before continuing. Stop at waist level.

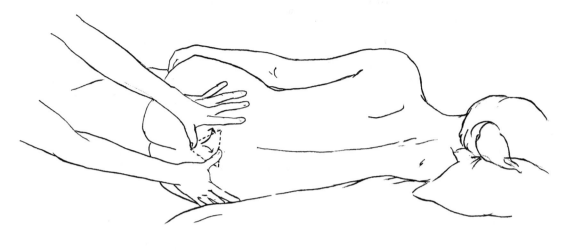

5.1

Alternate thumb circles on the sacrum during labor.

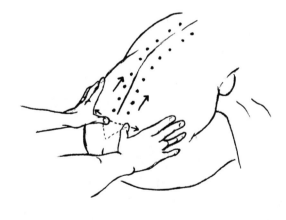

5.2

Pressure points along the spine and pelvis during labor.

4. Using your thumbs, outline the pelvis, starting from the sacrum and moving outward in one-inch increments until you reach the sides of her hip. At the center of her buttock, press in deeply (see illustration 5.3). Work with her breathing, pressing as she exhales and releasing as she inhales. Repeat three times.

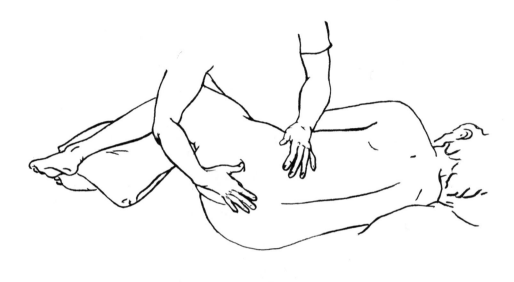

5.3

Pressure point in the center of the buttock.

5. Place the heel of your palm directly on her sacrum, supporting her shoulder with your other hand. Vibrate deeply into the bone for ten seconds (see illustration 5.4). Repeat two more times.

6. Complete the massage with a full effleurage from sacrum up and around her shoulders.

UPPER BACK: This treatment can also be done in a side-lying position, although the mother will have to turn to her other

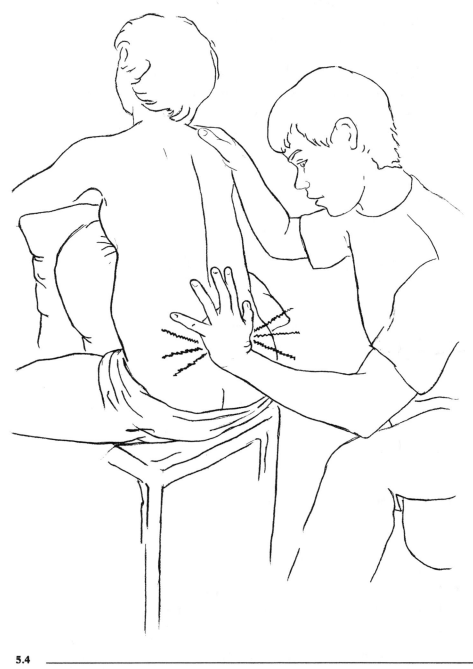

5.4

Vibration of the sacrum during labor.

side for maximum benefit. A seated position offers better access
to the entire back at one time.

1. Effleurage the full length of her back, from the sacrum up and
   around her shoulders, three times (see illustration 5.5). Continue massaging around her shoulders.

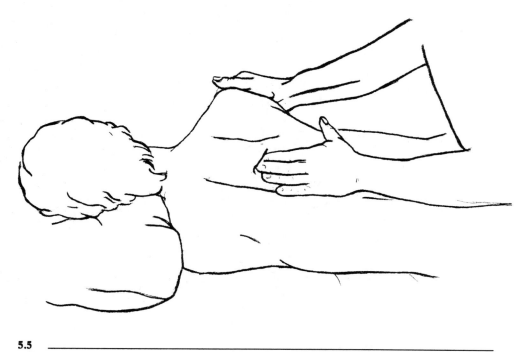

5.5

Effleurage of the back in a side-lying position.

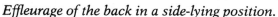

2. Using alternate thumb circles, massage along one shoulder
   blade at a time, concentrating on particularly sensitive areas.

3. Massage the top of her shoulders with both hands up to her
   neck and back down again. Press the point in the middle of
   her shoulders (see illustration 5.6). Have the mother drop her

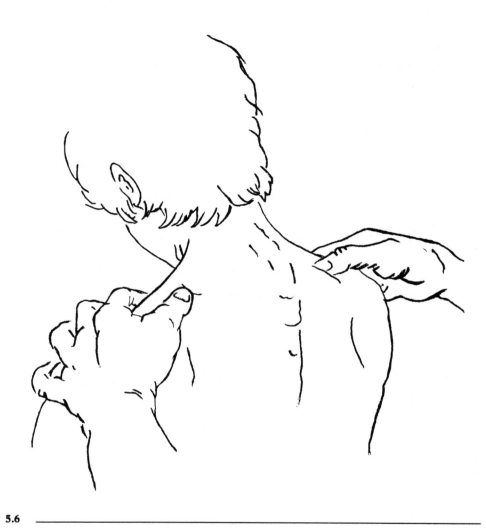

5.6

Pressure points in the middle of the shoulders.

head into one of your hands and squeeze the muscles in the back of her neck.

4. Repeat the full back effleurage several more times. Repeat this treatment on the other side if she was side-lying.

ABDOMINAL MASSAGE: A general, clockwise massage of the abdomen often brings welcome relief between labor contractions. The mother can be lying on her back, propped up with pillows under her head and knees, or in a side-lying position (see illustration 5.7).

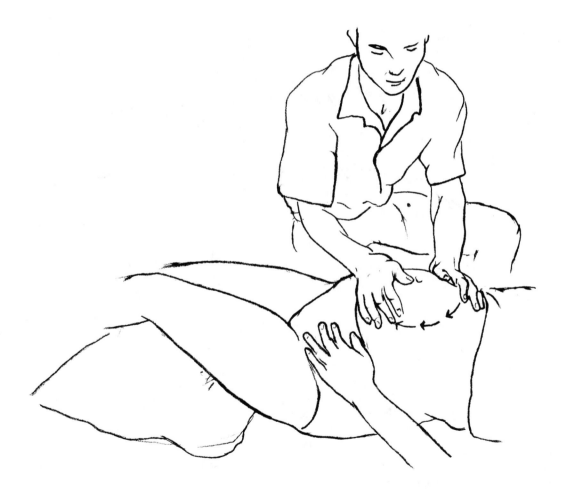

5.7

Clockwise massage of the abdomen.

L E G   M A S S A G E : Along with the back and abdomen, the legs get very tense during labor (and the feet often get cold, so remember to bring a pair of socks). General massage, consisting of effleurage of the legs and feet, helps to relax the muscles and reduce the pain. Several effleurage strokes on the front and back of her legs, from foot to hip, are very relaxing and beneficial. Foot massage will stimulate many reflex points, bringing about an easier labor.

L A B O R   P O I N T S : In addition to general massage, some Shiatsu and reflexology points are very powerful and can speed up labor and reduce pain. Up until this time in the pregnancy, use of these points is contraindicated. As a matter of fact, they are so powerful that uterine contractions and staining may occur if they are used in the early trimesters of pregnancy, so you are urged not to use these reflex points until labor actually begins.

1. Spleen 6 is approximately three inches above the inside ankle-bone, under the ridge of the shinbone (see illustration 5.8). When you locate the "button," press both legs with your thumbs. The mother will certainly acknowledge when you are on the correct spot. Hold for ten seconds and release. Repeat a total of three times.

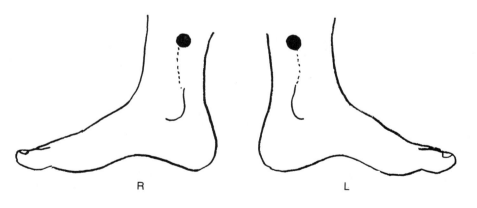

R   L

5.8

The Spleen 6 Shiatsu point is approximately three fingers width above the inner ankle.

2. The reflex points to the ovaries and uterus are under the anklebones in the center of the heel (see illustrations 5.9a and 5.9b). Squeeze them together, both feet at the same time, using thumbs and middle fingers. Hold for ten seconds and release. Repeat a total of three times.

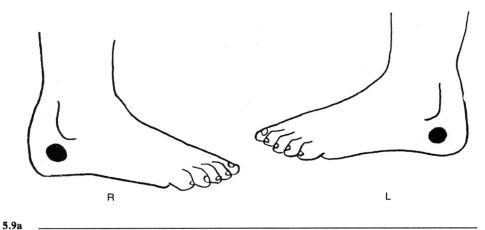

5.9a

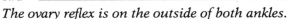

The ovary reflex is on the outside of both ankles.

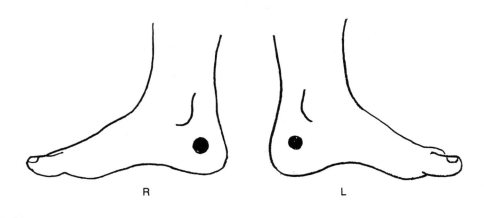

5.9b

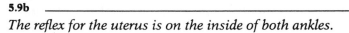

The reflex for the uterus is on the inside of both ankles.

FOR PROLONGED LABOR: Stimulation of the reflex points of the hands (along with the Spleen 6 point and ovary/uterus reflex points on the feet) during labor can help speed up the birthing process. Get several strong plastic or metal hair-combs (extras in case they break). Hold them in each hand so that the mother's fingertips support the edge and her palms receive the pressure from the teeth (see illustration 5.10). During your contractions, press the combs into the palms, alternating the position to stimulate all the reflexes in your hands.

Walking around will encourage labor. A general leg massage, between contractions, will relax your legs and help to stimulate labor. It is also important to do things that calm and relax you, such as bathing or meditating. Being anxious prompts adrenaline secretion, which sabotages oxytocin production, thus slowing down labor.

5.10

In cases of prolonged labor, press the combs into your palms with each contraction.

Trembling and/or shaking can occur at different times during and after labor. While placing your hands on her arms or legs may not stop the trembling, it does offer comfort and support and has a grounding effect. Or you can squeeze the inner arches of both feet, which may reduce the shaking considerably (see illustration 5.11).

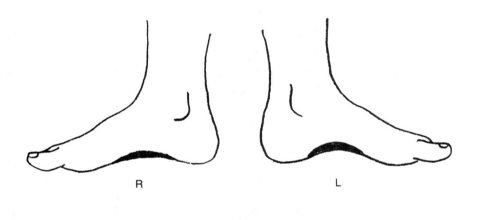

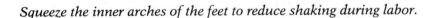

5.11

Squeeze the inner arches of the feet to reduce shaking during labor.

CHAPTER 6

POSTPARTUM
MASSAGE

*T*he six-week postpartum period is a recovery time when your body returns to normal. Your hormonal balance is reestablished, and the uterus involutes—that is, returns to its prepregnancy size. Fatigue is a common complaint, and many women experience "postpartum blues" for a few days or for as long as a few weeks. Adequate rest, proper nutrition, plenty of fluids, support, and massage help you to readjust and heal quickly.

There are some normal physical signs of the postpartum period that reflect the hormonal changes you are undergoing:

• Heavy and frequent urination.

• Increased perspiration.

• Contracted and firm uterus to prevent blood loss.

• Lochia is produced. This is a normal vaginal discharge resembling the menstrual flow for the first few days after birthing and then changing to a lighter red. It finally becomes a yellow or white discharge two weeks or so after the baby is born.

• Afterpains are experienced. These are contractions of

97

the uterus as it returns to its prepregnancy condition. Afterpains can be heightened by nursing, which speeds up the healing.

• A general soreness and stiffness from labor.

The perineum can be helped by the frequent application of ice packs for the first twenty-four hours or longer to reduce soreness and swelling. Hemorrhoids, which may have developed during labor, can be helped by the same massage techniques found in Chapter 2. The reflex points on the heels (see illustration 6.1) should be pressed at fifteen- to thirty-second intervals for five minutes. Remember to stimulate the colon reflex points for an unstrained bowel movement. The Shiatsu point on the top of the head also helps to treat hemorrhoids (see illustration 6.2).

Kegel exercises (see Chapter 4), which help restore tonicity to the perineal area, will also bring the blood away from the engorged pelvic veins. A cold sitz bath—up to four inches of clear

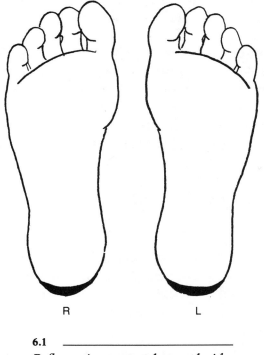

6.1

Reflex point to treat hemorrhoids.

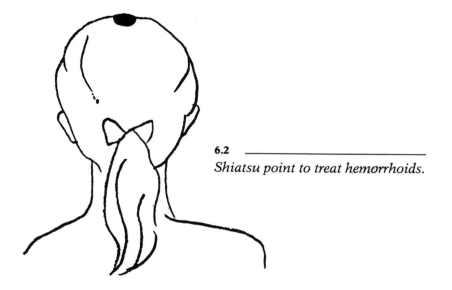

6.2
Shiatsu point to treat hemorrhoids.

water—is beneficial in shrinking the hemorrhoids. You can also apply lemon juice or witch hazel directly to the area.

Other common discomforts of the postpartum period are similar to those you might have experienced during pregnancy. The treatments for many of these conditions, which include abdominal weakness, backaches, breast soreness, constipation and heartburn, fatigue, headaches, and muscle soreness, can be found in Chapter 2.

Returning to your normal exercise regime will depend on your fitness before and during pregnancy, your body's condition after the birth, complications you might have experienced, and your own sense of how you feel. Discuss this with your doctor or health care provider before exercising again. Remember to begin slowly and cautiously. You will get stronger faster if you are careful about reentry into physical activity.

POSTPARTUM BLUES AND DEPRESSION

Postpartum blues are experienced by 60 percent of women within the first ten days of delivery. They are expressed by mood swings, tearfulness, poor concentration, anxiety, irritation, and even despondency. The blues often disappear after milk letdown happens, usually by the fourth day after delivery, and hormonal equilibrium is restored to prepregnancy levels. Recovery is spontaneous, and there are no relapses.

Postpartum depression differs in duration and severity. It affects only 10 percent of women and usually doesn't become evident until after the new mother returns home. The symptoms are similar to the blues, but can also include an inability to cope with the infant, increased anxiety without tears, and difficulty eating and/or sleeping. The postpartum depression can last for several months if not treated professionally.

Many factors can contribute to these depressed feelings, often referred to as the fourth trimester of pregnancy. The physiological, emotional, familial, social, and psychological changes that the new mother and father experience are profound stress factors. This is another transition stage, which requires love, patience, compassion, and understanding to overcome.

POSTPARTUM MASSAGE

One of the most important and universally accepted recovery procedures immediately after birth in the tribal world was massage. In the Philippines, massage was used throughout labor and postpartum to stimulate uterine involution. In the Maikal Hills of India, the birth attendant oiled her own head and rubbed it against the standing new mother's belly until all the blood came out. In Tahiti, the mother kneaded her own abdomen while bathing in the sea as her husband pressed his foot against her to stimulate further expulsion of birth materials.

The new mother can expedite involution of her uterus by massaging her abdomen in a clockwise, circular direction every four hours (see illustration 6.3). This will result in an increase of bleeding during or immediately after the procedure as lochia is secreted with the uterine contractions. This indicates an effective massage. The new mother should continue the massage until the color of the lochia discharge is pale, usually up to two weeks.

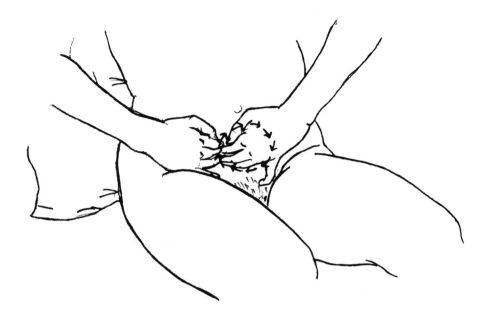

6.3

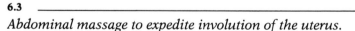

Abdominal massage to expedite involution of the uterus.

A full body massage (see Chapter 3) offers relief from the aches and pains of muscle soreness, wards off fatigue, and promotes rapid healing. The father should include two Shiatsu points in his treatment of the mother's lower back; one is at the base of the sacrum, and the other on the vertebra just below waist level (see illustration 6.4). Hold each point for fifteen seconds and release. Repeat two more times.

HERBS: Red raspberry leaf tea should continue to be consumed throughout the day. Health food stores have herbal commercial teas that are specifically for pregnancy and postpartum recovery.

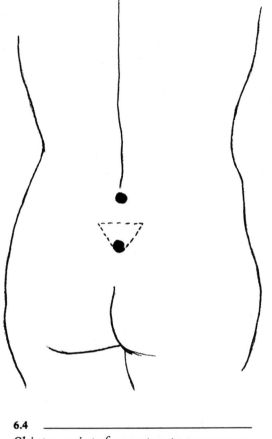

Shiatsu points for postpartum massage.

For women who have had C-sections, a warm ginger compress (see the section on breast soreness in Chapter 2) applied from the navel to the stitches promotes rapid healing. Wait until the wound has closed before treating the scar.

In Java, the abdomen of the new mother was massaged for the first five days and then intermittently for the next month. Abdominal binding was also a common practice in traditional cultures to restore the mother's shape. Many tribes honored the new mother by binding her with strips of cloth or ropes.

CHAPTER 7

NURSING

*L*actation begins when your breasts start to secrete colostrum prior to labor. Your milk doesn't actually let down for another few days, usually by the fourth day after birthing. Milk flow could be delayed due to a heavily medicated birth, if you are ill, or due to stress.

Oxytocin and prolactin are released as the baby sucks, signaling the release of milk from the milk glands in your breasts. Both colostrum and breast milk are produced by small glands deep in the breasts. These alveoli increase in number and size during pregnancy. A few days after having the baby, the milk is collected in the milk sinuses under the areola. This milk is called foremilk and is the first milk the baby drinks at each feeding. It is high in protein and low in fat.

As the baby suckles, the mother's brain sends signals to the pituitary gland, and oxytocin is released. This hormone causes the cells around the alveoli to contract and squeeze the milk into the duct system and out through the openings in the nipples. This is what is commonly known as milk letdown. The milk from the letdown, called hindmilk, is high in fat and makes up two thirds of the breast milk the baby will drink at each feeding.

Human milk is ideal for the infant. It is rich in nutrients and antibodies, protects against tooth decay, reduces the chance of your child having an allergic reaction to formulas, is high in iron, is easy to digest, and doesn't require preparation. For the mother, nursing offers emotional fulfillment, helps heal the uterus more quickly, and uses up extra body fat stored for this purpose.

MASSAGE FOR NURSING

The Modoc of California and women in parts of Guam and Africa employed breast massage to stimulate milk flow.

A full body massage will reduce any stress that might sabotage milk letdown. See Chapter 3 for discussion of a full body massage. The massage you did for breast soreness (see Chapter 2) will help stimulate milk letdown and offer relief in cases of engorgement.

The massage can be self-administered or performed by your partner. Work lightly and carefully, and avoid any direct nipple contact.

1. Using oil or cream, lightly circle around both breasts. Keep your pressure light and even.

2. Circle around one breast. With your fingertips, make tiny circles on the breast (see illustration 7.1). Repeat on the other breast.

3. Place both hands flat on either side on one breast, and slowly slide outward from the areola (see illustration 7.2). Alter the hand position around the breast. Repeat on the other breast.

4. Press the point in the middle of the shoulder (see illustration 7.3). Hold for fifteen seconds, and repeat two more times. This point should be avoided while pregnant but may be used now to stimulate milk flow.

For a lack of milk, include the Shiatsu point between the sixth and seventh ribs, at nipple level on the sternum.

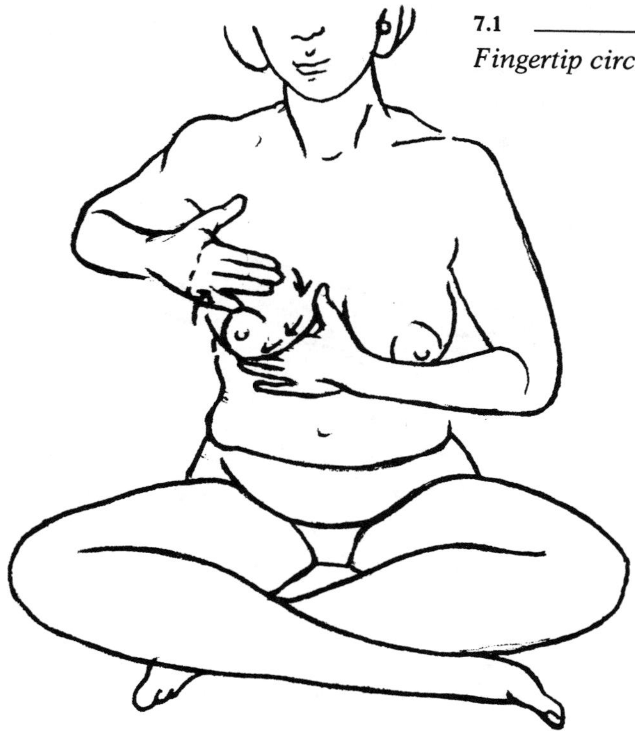

7.1

Fingertip circles around each breast.

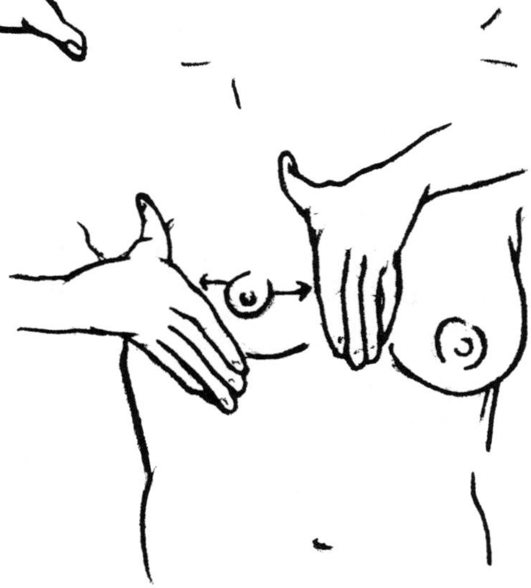

7.2

Slide outward from areola.

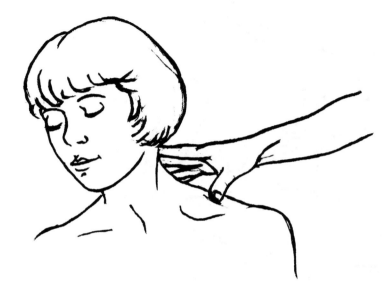

Shiatsu point in the middle of the shoulder to stimulate lactation.

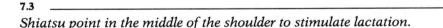

HERBS: Blessed thistle tea is a wonderful tea for nursing mothers. You may also drink peppermint tea. Be sure to drink extra fluids, including water with lemon.

TO DECREASE MILK FLOW

For those women who cannot or prefer not to nurse, use ice packs on your breasts to inhibit milk flow. One teaspoonful each of sage and alfalfa teas in one cup of water can be consumed often.

MASTITIS WHILE NURSING: Make a compress of equal parts of lavender oil, geranium oil, and rose oil in one quart of hot water. Let it cool, and apply the compress to your breasts for 15 minutes. Continue nursing even though the infection is present. You will heal faster.

Be sure to wash yourself after any treatment to your breasts before you nurse.

CHAPTER 8

INFANT MASSAGE

*I*t's a natural instinct to fondle, cuddle, and caress your baby. Our tribal foremothers cared for their children in resourceful and simplistic ways that produced healthy, well-bred children who were able to cope successfully against some of nature's harshest living conditions. It promoted closeness for the tribe, which was often vital for survival.

The Ibo of Nigeria sit on the floor and dip a fibrous loofah sponge into an herbal mixture. Then the mother vigorously rubs her baby with the wet loofah. She presses the bones of the skull together and massages the spine and limbs. When the treatment is finished, the mother blows forcefully into the eyes, nostrils, mouth, and ears of the baby. The child, dripping wet, is put down to rest beside the fire, often on a bare floor or a banana leaf.

Babies need touch to survive. The benefits from the massage are just beginning to be studied and understood but seem to indicate long-lasting effects on the health, growth, development, and well-being of the baby.

Massage for the infant actually begins in utero, with uterine contractions. Labor contractions stimulate the child's skin, which in turn activates the autonomic nervous system, sending messages to the respiratory system signaling the baby's first task after birth: to breathe. Other internal systems are also prepared to help the baby function "on the outside" through cutaneous (skin) stimulation. Since we don't lick our newborns as other mammals do—vital to the life of those offspring—the longer human labor offers stimulation for the baby's organ systems.

Babies delivered through C-section don't get the cutaneous stimulation of the birth canal and benefit enormously from massage.

What are the benefits of massage to your baby?

• Bonding becomes stronger as love is exchanged and communicated through touch. This results in more loving, relaxed adults. Parental attachment becomes greater. Bonding has been an issue of great importance and debate recently. Massage contains all the essential elements of bonding: eye-to-eye contact, skin-to-skin contact, smiles, laughter, soothing sounds, cuddling, smell, response, and communication. Babies thrive on this interaction. Massage enhances all the characteristics of bonding. Love abounds and remains a lasting connection between child and parent.

• Massage helps the child's circulation.

• Massage stimulates internal organs.

• Massage helps relieve colic and intestinal gas.

• A study at the Rainbow Babies' and Children's Hospital in Cleveland, Ohio, showed that intellectual development is enhanced through early touch, raising language development, reading scores, and IQs.

• Massage reduces stress and helps the baby to cope better. Sleep is promoted.

• Massage exercises the child and teaches the child about his body.

• The baby's immune system is strengthened.

• There is faster weight gain and general well-being. Low-birth-weight babies benefit from infant massage by an increase in appetite.

• There is an increase in cardiac output. Massage promotes fuller and deeper respiration.

• Skin stimulation has been shown to increase endorphin output, decreasing pain and tension.

• Massage increases gentleness and friendliness and makes loving children develop into loving adults.

We cannot overlook the beneficial effects that infant massage has on the provider:

• Massaging the infant benefits the mother by enhancing the secretion of prolactin, essential for milk production. She is therefore more successful in breast feeding.

• The parents become more proficient and capable in their nurturing abilities.

• The relationship to the parent is strengthened, part of the bonding process.

• Massage provides a loving way to learn about your child. You will learn what pleases him and what is uncomfortable. A communication channel opens wide for you both.

• The father enjoys the same emotional fulfillment as the mother. The baby learns that the father can also offer physical and emotional support. The bonding between father and child through massage cannot be accomplished by any other parenting technique.

All the advantages that massage offers the adult are equally present in infant massage, and then some. By taking the time to massage your child, you are teaching love, respect, and caring.

Infant massage can begin when the baby is one month old. Daily massage is recommended. They generally last no longer than thirty minutes and are cherished respites from your normally hectic routine.

When the baby starts to crawl, you can massage less frequently—two or three times per week should suffice. Some children want the massages to continue until they are a lot more independent.

It's a good idea not to massage the baby immediately after a feeding. Find the time that works out best for you and the baby, and try to stick to it.

Some babies fall asleep during or immediately after the massage. It is most enjoyable to bathe the baby in warm water after the treatment. The relaxing effects of the massage stay longer as any residual tensions "wash away."

SUPPLIES

The most important factor to remember is keeping the baby warm and away from drafts. Heating the oil in the winter months is a good idea.

Find a quiet place, and sit on the floor. Cross your legs or stretch them in front of you, whichever is more comfortable.

The items you will need are:

• Massage oil. Cold-pressed vegetable oils are preferred. Almond or sesame oils found in health food stores are fine. You can add vitamins such as A, D, and E to the oil, for greater skin care. Natural oils will not irritate sensitive skin. Keep the oil in a spillproof plastic bottle to avoid accidents.

Our tribal foremothers knew that nutrients in the oil would be absorbed by the infant's delicate skin. A Kwakiutl baby of North America would be rubbed with olachin oil in cases of colds or constipation. This was the medicine drunk by adults with the same ailments. Other tribal people used oils rich in vitamins, such as vitamin D, which is not abundant in breast milk.

• A pillow covered with towels for the provider's legs is optional but offers more comfort.

• Extra towel and diapers. Babies have no bladder or bowel

control, and the relaxation enjoyed from the massage makes them empty their bladders.

• A warm blanket or change of clothes for the baby to wear after the massage or bath.

INFANT MASSAGE

Work gently. Slowly. Softly. Lovingly. A light touch in the first month is sufficient. After one month, a firmer pressure may be applied. Premature babies should be massaged once an ample amount of weight has been gained and the doctor has approved it.

Maintain eye contact. Talk quietly. Keep a rhythmic pace throughout the massage. Heed the baby's responses; they are his words. (At this point I want to apologize to all the girl babies receiving this massage. I am generically referring to the baby as "him" for convenience.)

Keep a few things in mind while you are working: You can spend as much time as you or the baby want on any area. If the baby responds favorably to a particular stroke, repeat it. Let instinct guide you, and let your baby give you the feedback.

"HELLO" STROKE

In Swedish massage, it is the nerve stroke. It's a very light stroke that glides over the body without pressure. For the baby, it signals the beginning and end of the massage.

1. With the baby on his back on your outstretched legs, or on a towel in front of you, look into his eyes and place both hands gently on his head. Lightly slide down his face, chest, hips, thighs, and all the way down to his toes (see illustration 8.1). Softly stretch out his legs as you glide on them. Talk to him. Your voice conveys love and gentleness, which is reflected in your touch.

2. Lift your hands and repeat the stroke, this time stretching his

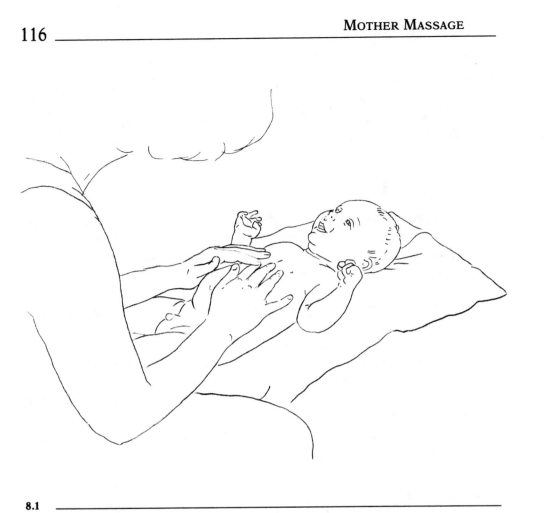

8.1 _____

"Hello" stroke. Lightly slide down from his head to his toes. Maintain eye contact.

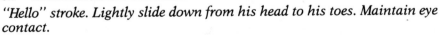

arms and fingers. Return to his chest and continue the stroke down to his toes.

If the baby offers resistance to the stretch, don't force it.

FACE

1. Warm a little bit of oil between your hands. Place the flats of your fingers in the center of the forehead and stretch out to the sides of his temples. Continue down the sides of his face and come together at the chin.

2. With your thumbs, trace his eyebrows from the bridge of his nose outward.

3. Still using your thumbs, stretch lightly and softly across his closed eyelids.

4. From the bridge of his nose, trace down his nose and pull out under his cheekbones (see illustration 8.2).

5. Make tiny circles on his jaw.

6. Massage his ears.

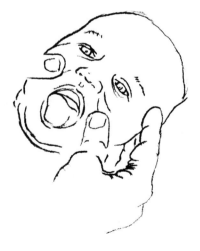

8.2

Trace down his nose and pull out under his cheekbones.

CHEST

1. Place your hands in the center of his chest and move slowly out to each side (see illustration 8.3). Keep your fingertips on his body, and circle back to your starting point.

2. Place your thumbs on his upper chest muscles and fan outward. If there is any chest congestion, light fingertip tapping on the breastbone and muscles of the chest will help bring up the phlegm.

3. Using the flats of your fingers, place them behind his ears and stroke down the sides of his neck across the top of his shoulders. Retrace the movement and repeat it.

4. Place your right hand on his right shoulder and cross diagonally to his left hip (see illustration 8.4). Follow this with the left hand on the left shoulder, crossing to his right hip. Repeat this "X" movement a few more times.

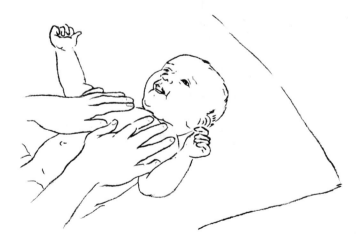

8.3

From the center of his chest, glide out to each side.

5. Repeat the "X" stroke and continue all the way down to the opposite leg and foot, stretching the limb as you stroke. Remember to keep eye contact and your rhythm at a steady pace.

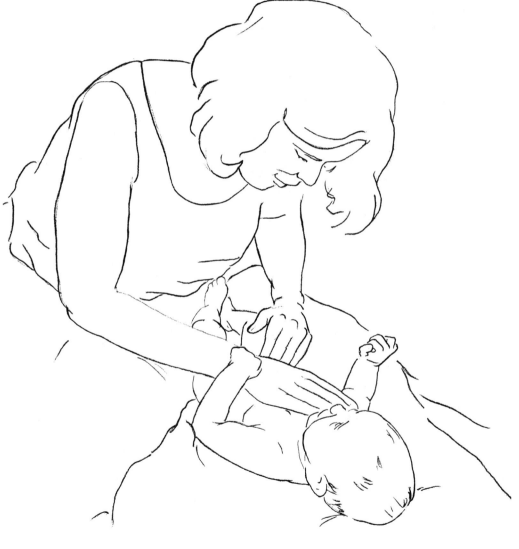

8.4

"X" stroke to opposite hips.

ABDOMEN

Massage of the abdomen is wonderful to release gas, relieve constipation, and for internal stimulation of the organs. Be sure the umbilical cord is completely healed before massaging his stomach. This treatment will help colicky babies.

Follow a clockwise direction. If your infant is uncomfortable or fidgety, it could be because of gas. Lighten the pressure and talk to him.

1. Place your warm, oiled hands on the baby's belly, on either side of the navel, and just remain there for a few moments.

2. With your left palm above the navel, the right palm on the opposite side beneath the navel, trace a clockwise pattern. Move both hands at the same time (see illustration 8.5). This is achieved by making opposing half circles. When your arms cross over each other, lift them and replace them at the same spot, using the other hand. Continue the circle. This action

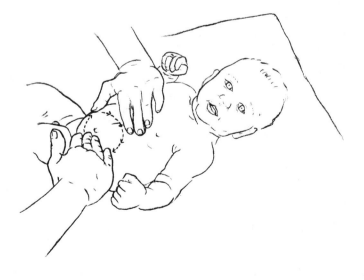

8.5 _____

Clockwise effleurage of baby's abdomen.

stimulates the peristaltic—wavelike—action of the intestines. (This is the same stroke you do for the mother or the father on the abdomen.)

3. One hand follows the other with this next stroke. From under his rib cage, stretch the abdomen downward, using the sides of your hand (see illustration 8.6).

4. If there is still some gas trapped and your baby is uncomfortable because of it, lift the baby's legs and let them rest against your stomach. You might have to hold them in place. With your free hand, trace a circle around his stomach, starting from the lower left corner. Stay approximately 1 to 1½ inches from his navel while making the circle.

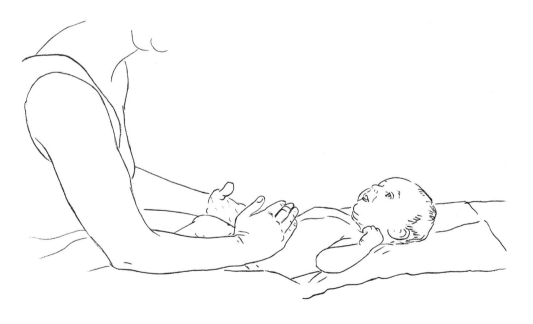

8.6

Alternate hand stroke of abdomen. If your baby still has gas, lift his legs and rest them against your stomach. Continue the stroke. Be sure your baby is covered with a diaper.

ARMS

1. Turn your baby to one side. Hold his arm extended, and massage with a long stroke from shoulder to hand (see illustration 8.7). Repeat with your other hand.

2. Using both hands, twist his arms in opposite directions from his shoulder to his wrist and back to his shoulder (see illustration 8.8).

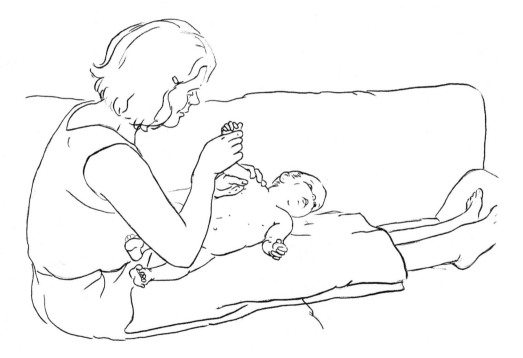

8.7

Stroke his arm from shoulder to hand.

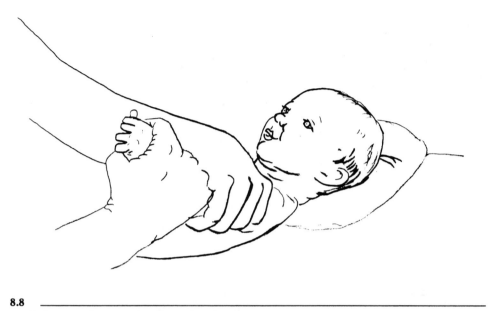

8.8

Lightly twist his arm in opposite directions.

3. Open his hand with your thumbs and crisscross his palm. Follow this with alternate thumb circles. Run your thumb up each finger, carefully stretching them.

4. Gently turn him over and repeat the same sequence on the other arm.

LEGS

1. The leg massage follows the same pattern as the arms, except that your baby can relax comfortably on his back once again. Remember to maintain eye contact as much as possible. Lift one leg and alternately massage with a long stroke from his hip to his foot (see illustration 8.9). Repeat with your other hand.

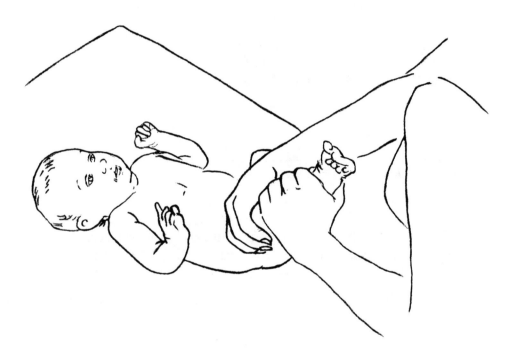

8.9

Alternate hand stroke of the leg. Remember to smile at, talk to, and look at your baby.

2. Twist his leg in opposing directions from hip to foot and back to hip.

3. Open his foot with your thumbs and crisscross his sole (see illustration 8.10). Follow this with alternate circles. Run your thumb up each toe, carefully stretching them. Flex the ankle. Repeat the same sequence on the other leg.

4. When you have completed with both legs, finish the massage with a gentle nerve stroke, from his head to his toes.

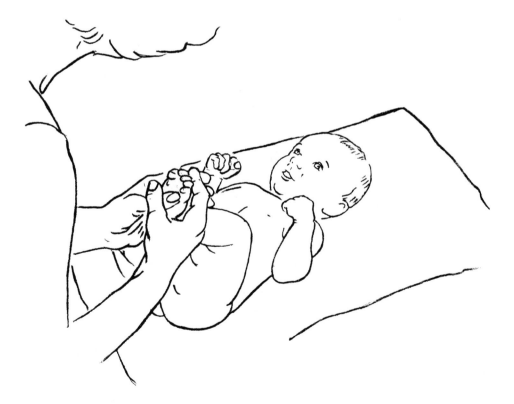

8.10

Crisscross stroke on his foot.

BACK

1. Turn him over and place him across your legs. A nerve stroke from the top of his head to his toes says "hello." Then cross his back with gliding strokes, your hands working opposite each other, from his neck to his buttocks and back to his neck. You are transversing his spine.

2. Secure one hand on his buttocks and stroke up and down his back (see illustration 8.11).

3. Make wide circles around each shoulder, tracing each shoulder blade.

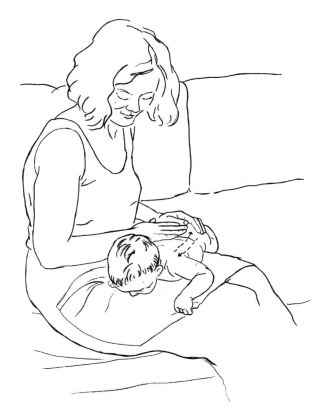

8.11 ————————————————————

Secure one hand on his buttocks and stroke up and down his back.

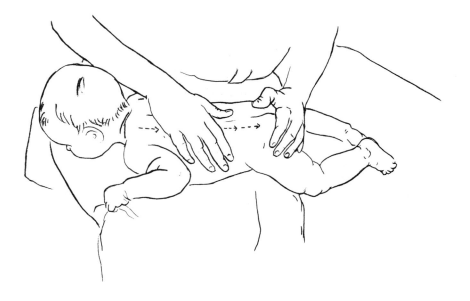

8.12

Support his buttocks and stroke down his back. Avoid pressure on his delicate spine.

4. Support his buttocks and slowly work down his spine with your other hand. Avoid direct pressure to his spine (see illustration 8.12). Repeat this stroke three times.

5. Hold the baby's ankles and gently extend his legs. Stroke down from his neck, over his buttocks to his heels (see illustration 8.13).

6. Slowly release his legs and make light, alternate circles on his sacrum with your thumbs.

7. End the massage with several light nerve strokes, from head to toe.

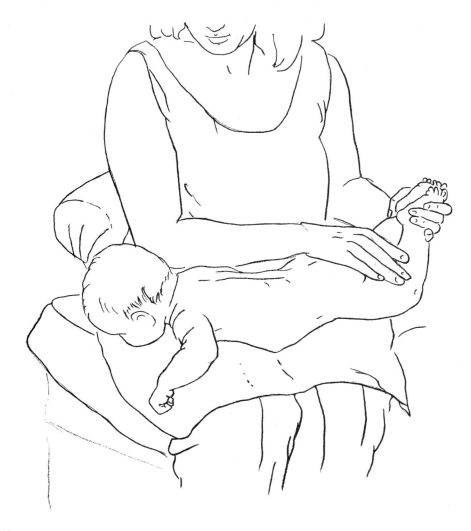

8.13

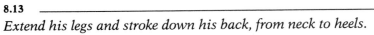

Extend his legs and stroke down his back, from neck to heels.

STRETCHES

Turn the baby on his back again. Make eye contact. Talk to him.

The stretches should be done slowly and gently. They are exercises that will strengthen his muscles, provide flexibility to his joints, teach him about his body, and offer a lot of pleasure.

1. Arm stretch. Take each of the baby's hands and cross them over his chest. Then open his arms wide and out to the sides. Cross over his chest again and then bring his arms over his head (see illustration 8.14). Bring them to his sides and release them.

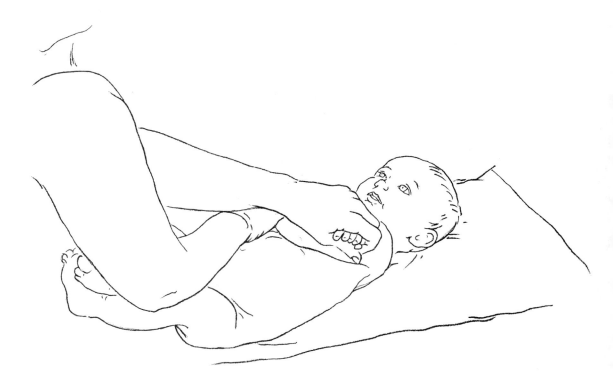

8.14

Arm stretch. Cross his arms over his chest. Open them wide out to his sides. Cross his chest again and stretch them over his head.

2. Arm-leg stretch. Take one arm and the opposite leg and bring them together. Stretch them out (see illustration 8.15). Repeat two more times. Do the same stretch with his other limbs.

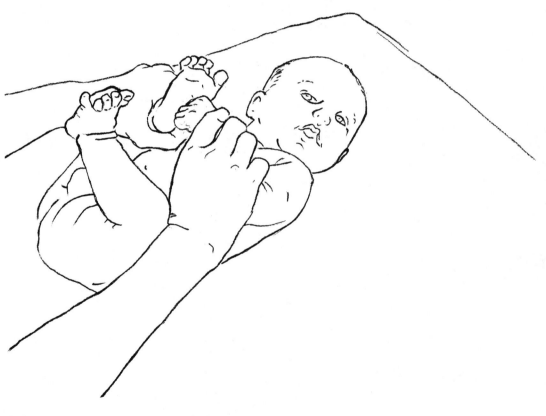

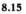

8.15 _____

Arm-leg stretch. Bring one arm and his opposite leg together. Stretch them out and repeat with the other limbs.

3. Leg stretch. Take his feet and cross his legs over his abdomen. Carefully stretch them out (see illustration 8.16). Repeat two more times.

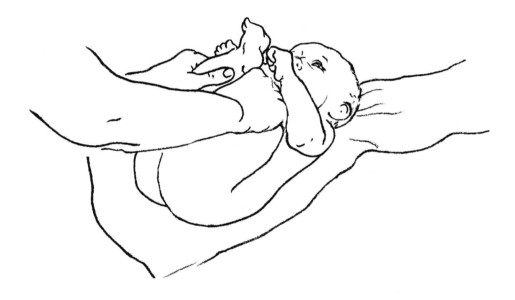

8.16

Leg stretch. Cross his legs over his abdomen. Carefully stretch them out.

CHAPTER 9

REFLEXOLOGY AND SHIATSU QUICK REFERENCE TABLE

DISCOMFORT	ILLUSTRATION	TREATMENT
Allergies and sinus congestion	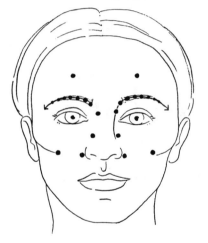	Hold each point for thirty seconds.
Allergies and sinus congestion	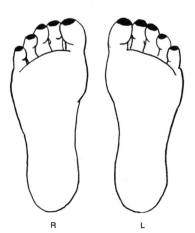	Hold each point for thirty seconds.

DISCOMFORT	ILLUSTRATION	TREATMENT
Anemia	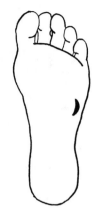	The reflex point for the treatment of anemia is found on the left foot only. Hold the point until any tenderness or soreness disappears.
Backaches	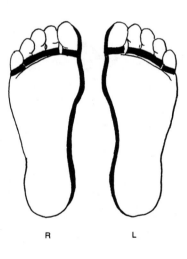	Massage the points until the soreness disappears.
	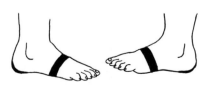	Massage the points until the soreness disappears.

DISCOMFORT	ILLUSTRATION	TREATMENT
Breast soreness		Hold the points until the soreness disappears.
Constipation and heartburn	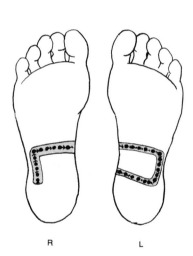	Starting with the right foot, press the points along the intestinal reflex, holding each point for thirty seconds.
Hemorrhoids	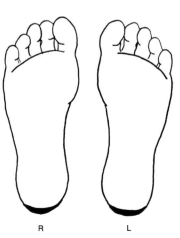	Press the reflex point for fifteen to thirty seconds. Release. Treat each foot for five minutes.

DISCOMFORT	ILLUSTRATION	TREATMENT

Hemorrhoids

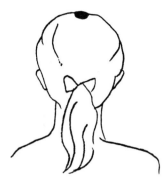

Press three times for fifteen seconds.

Labor

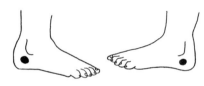

Squeeze the uterus/ ovary reflexes of both feet at the same time. Hold for ten seconds. Release. Repeat a total of three times.

Squeeze the uterus/ ovary reflexes of both feet at the same time. Hold for ten seconds. Release. Repeat a total of three times.

DISCOMFORT	ILLUSTRATION	TREATMENT

Labor

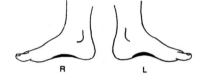

Press the Spleen 6 Shiatsu point for ten seconds. Release. Repeat a total of three times.

Squeeze the arches of the feet during labor to reduce shaking.

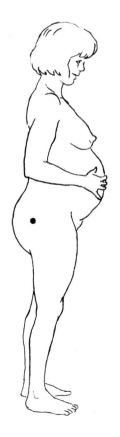

Press in deeply on exhalation and release on inhalation. Repeat three times.

DISCOMFORT	ILLUSTRATION	TREATMENT

Postpartum

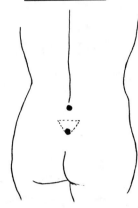

Hold each point for fifteen seconds. Release. Repeat a total of three times.

Sciatica

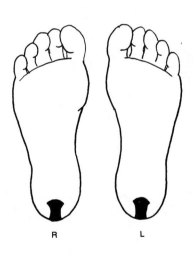

Hold each point for fifteen seconds. Release for five seconds. Repeat a total of three times.

DISCOMFORT	ILLUSTRATION	TREATMENT
Sciatica	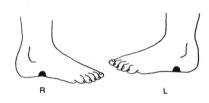	Hold each point for fifteen seconds. Release for five seconds. Repeat a total of three times.
		Hold each point for fifteen seconds. Release for five seconds. Repeat a total of three times.

CHAPTER 10

HERBAL REMEDY QUICK REFERENCE TABLE

*T*his table summarizes the herbal treatments listed in this book, as well as some nutritional advice. All the aromatic oils are essential oils found in herb or health food stores.

DISCOMFORT	REMEDY
Allergies, sinus congestion	Inhale two to three drops of eucalyptus oil in warm water.
Anemia	Dandelion tea; yellow dock tea
Backaches	Massage oil: ten drops of juniper oil, six drops of lavender oil, and eight drops of rosemary oil in two fluid ounces of vegetable oil
Breast soreness	Warm ginger compress for thirty minutes
Cesarean scars	Warm ginger compress

DISCOMFORT	REMEDY
Charley horse—leg cramps	Diet rich in calcium
Edema	Soak hands and feet in Epsom salts: four cups of boiling water and two cups of Epsom salts in bathwater; vitamin B_6
Headaches	Nettle tea, three tablespoons to one cup; yerba santa tea, one teaspoon to one cup
Heartburn	Take two to three drops on the tongue of peppermint, rose, or sandalwood oils.
Hemorrhoids	Witch hazel; lemon juice; vitamin E; vitamin B_6 orally
Insomnia	One cup of hops tea; one cup of scullcap tea; one cup of chamomile tea
Labor massage oil	Twelve drops of clary sage oil, five drops of rose oil, and five drops of ylang-ylang in two fluid ounces of vegetable oil
Mastitis	Warm compress of equal parts of lavender oil, geranium oil, and rose oil in one quart of water
Morning sickness	Red raspberry leaf tea; peppermint tea
Nursing	Blessed thistle tea; peppermint tea
Perineum care	Sitz bath of two drops of cypress oil and four drops of lavender oil in shallow bath

DISCOMFORT	REMEDY
Postpartum care	Red raspberry leaf tea
Sore nipples	Two drops of rose oil in one ounce of sweet almond oil
Stretch marks	Vitamin E on marks; massage oil of twenty-five drops of lavender oil and five drops of neroli oil (optional) in two ounces of wheat germ oil
Varicose veins	Vitamin C, 100 milligrams; vitamin E, 600 I.U.

Expectant Mother's and Developing Baby's Growth

MOTHER: YOUR FIRST TRIMESTER

Although no two pregnancies are ever alike, there are basic physical changes that are normal in all pregnancies. These changes begin almost immediately after conception. After all, your body has to adapt itself to support the new life.

During the first three months, extra amounts of estrogen, the female hormone, are released. Morning sickness and nausea are often caused by this sudden hormonal increase. Sometimes a thickening can be felt throughout your body (waistbands start to get tight early on), and a sensitivity in your breasts can be felt as early as two weeks after conception. Perhaps you notice a change of pigmentation, especially around the nipples. This is also due to the extra amounts of hormones.

Uterine cramping may be felt, although this is generally most noticeable in the third trimester. These early cramps are called Braxton-Hicks contractions. They are caused by your uterus stretching and preparing itself for the pregnancy. It is exercising, getting into shape. By the eighth week, your uterus is four inches long and the placenta takes up a third of the womb. At ten weeks this organ weighs seven ounces, one to three ounces of which is amniotic fluid.

Light-headedness and fainting may occur and can be caused by a drop in normal blood pressure. Eating frequent but small meals throughout the day may prevent this by raising your blood sugar.

The joints between the pelvic bones widen and are movable by the end of the first trimester. The hormone relaxin is responsible for this change.

Fatigue is not an uncommon occurrence at the onset of pregnancy. Once again, it is a natural effect of the hormones. Make sure that your diet is well balanced; this will help overcome the bouts of fatigue.

Expect to gain about three pounds during your first trimester.

BABY: THE FIRST TRIMESTER

Ten days after conception: The embryo has moved down the Fallopian tube and implanted itself in the wall of your uterus (womb), where it will stay, be nourished, and grow for the next nine months.

Second week: Hundreds of cells are dividing quickly. A basic heart is developing. The embryo begins to elongate. It is less than one-tenth inch long and plate-shaped.

Third week: The embryo attaches itself to the placenta, which will supply all the life-sustaining nourishment. The initial brain division is visible, and the limbs are now short buds.

Fourth week: The eyes begin to develop. The heart separates into right and left halves and is beating by the twenty-fifth day. Lungs begin to develop, and there is the beginning of a circulatory system, simple kidneys, a liver, and a digestive tract. The embryo has its distinctive fetal curl, and the face is starting to form. It is one-quarter inch long and ten thousand times larger than the egg from which it was fertilized.

Fifth week (second month): The feet and hands begin to form. The collarbone and lower jaw start to ossify (become bone). The ears and nose begin to develop, and the heart is now pumping sixty-five times per minute.

Sixth week: The skeleton is complete. Major organs are visible and growing rapidly. Leg buds develop as the outlines of fingers and toes begin to appear. The nose can be seen, and the eyelids are forming. The embryo is one-half to three-quarters inch long.

Seventh week: Muscles start to form. More bones solidify. The stomach begins to make digestive juices, the liver makes blood cells, and the kidneys begin to function. Eye lenses form. The embryo can move its hands and fingers. The ears develop together, and the first buds of teeth appear. The embryo is now three-quarters to one inch long.

Eighth week: Limbs are well defined, and finger- and foot-prints appear. Bones continue to ossify. The head is rather large, and the neck is clearly visible. The embryo is one inch long and weighs one-thirtieth ounce.

Ninth week (third month): The halves of the hard palate on the roof of the mouth unite. The gallbladder is visible. The embryo can now move within the uterus. Nails begin to grow, and the eyelids close for the first time. The external sex organs are discernible, while the internal sex organs are developing. The embryo can frown, swallow, and suck its thumb. Vocal cords are completed, and urination begins. The embryo and placenta are about equal in size at the end of the first trimester. After ten weeks, the embryo is two inches long. After eleven weeks it is two and a half inches long, and by the twelfth week, three inches. It weighs one ounce.

MOTHER: YOUR SECOND TRIMESTER

During the second trimester, your body has adjusted to the hormonal changes, and the nausea usually ceases. Fetal movement can be felt and the heartbeat heard through a special instrument called a fetal scope. If a woman is thirty-five years or older, an amniocentesis is usually performed during the fourth month. It is a relatively safe procedure wherein a long needle is inserted through the expectant mother's abdominal wall into the amniotic sac. Fluid is extracted and tested for the presence of any genetic defects in the fetus.

Your uterus grows a lot during the second trimester and reaches to your navel by the fifth month. Weight gain is apparent, and as much as ten pounds can be gained by the end of the sixth month. You will begin to show during this trimester.

Maternal breathing starts to become shallow as the lungs are depressed by the diaphragm. Breathing exercises often help, and lifting the arms over your head gives more breathing space.

As the fetus continues to develop, some women experience tingling sensations in their extremities because so much blood is being rerouted to nourish the placenta.

Your lower back might ache due to the strain of weight displacement as your child grows larger. Proper posture and body mechanics (and flat shoes!) are especially important from this time to the end of pregnancy.

Anytime from the fifth month on, colostrum, a yellowish fluid that will be the child's first food, may be produced by the mammary glands in your breasts. Natural fiber shields or pads will absorb any leaking fluid.

BABY: THE SECOND TRIMESTER

Fourth month: Fat under the skin develops. The nails become hard, and nipples appear. Tonsils can be seen, and the sensory organs are completely formed. The fetus (as it is now called) can turn inside the uterus. At four and a half months, the fetus is six inches long and weighs four ounces. The mouth and lips are completely shaped, and eyebrows and lashes grow. The fetus has sleeping and waking cycles and can see, although the eyes are still closed.

Fifth month: The germs of permanent teeth appear in the jaws. Hair grows on the head. The base of the tongue and lymphatic glands are evident. The fetus can grip with its hands now. A hairy growth called lanugo appears on the arms, legs, and back. Fetal movement, called quickening, is felt. It is now ten to twelve inches long and weighs eight ounces to one pound. The fetus is growing quickly.

Sixth month: The spine begins to ossify. The free borders of the nails project from the skin. Most of the lanugo disappears, although a trace may remain on a newborn baby. The skin is red, wrinkled, and covered with a protective coating called vernix caseosa, which stays on the baby even after it is born. The umbilical cord reaches maximum length at this time. The fetus is eleven to fourteen inches long and weighs one to two pounds.

MOTHER: YOUR THIRD TRIMESTER

During the last trimester, weight gain continues. Calcium which is stored in the body in your teeth and bones, is absorbed by the fetus in large quantities as it continues to grow. It is important that you replace this mineral to meet your baby's demand and to avert leg cramps or cavities.

Swelling of the feet (edema), headaches, sinus congestion, and fatigue are not uncommon during the final trimester. Eat adequate amounts of protein to minimize fatigue and reduce swelling of the extremities.

The fatty tissues in your breasts increase and your breasts become heavy, tender, and sensitive. Blue veins surface on your chest and breasts as the blood supply increases and blood vessels enlarge.

Backaches are especially common. Constipation and gas occur because your enlarged uterus compresses the intestines, which slows digestion. Iron supplements may also cause constipation. The stretch marks that appear may be reduced by applying vitamin E or special oils to the affected areas. General massage, or any type of stress-reducing treatment, also helps to slow down the stretch mark process.

There is an increase in vaginal discharge throughout the

entire pregnancy but predominantly in the final trimester. It is caused by the increase in the supply of blood and hormones to the area. You may notice that you are very warm, or even hot, at times during the last few months. Your bone marrow is producing more blood cells, which increases your total blood volume by 30 to 50 percent. As a result, more iron is needed. Your heart changes position and gets slightly larger to accommodate the demand.

Body weight is increased by ten to twelve pounds, bringing the total recommended healthy weight gain to twenty-four to thirty pounds.

By the end of the pregnancy, your uterus will have increased its size five to six times, its weight twenty times and its capacity a thousand times. The uterus finally grows to fourteen inches long and weighs two and a quarter pounds, while the placenta weighs one and a half pounds at term. Your uterus is now seven to nine inches in diameter.

As birth nears, milk glands start to produce colostrum, and the hormones prepare for the first contractions of labor.

BABY: THE THIRD TRIMESTER

Seventh month: There is continued growth and movement. All important physiological systems are developed, and the fetus settles in a head-down position, getting ready for birth. It is sixteen inches long.

Eighth month: The fetus has smooth skin and is growing fatter. It is eighteen inches long and weighs five pounds.

Ninth month: The heart is pumping six hundred pints of blood a day. The eyelids open and close. The skin is still covered with vernix caseosa. There is continued growth. At the end of the nine months, the baby weighs seven to eight pounds. The baby drops into the pelvis, and the head fits into the birth position.

The weight of the fertilized egg has been increased five billion times. One single cell has divided into two hundred million cells.

A child is born.

Nutritional Daily Requirements

The United States Recommended Daily Allowances (USRDA 1986) for pregnant and lactating women are as follows:

KCal.	2,500
Vitamin A	8,000 I.U.
Thiamine (B_1)	1.7 mg.
Riboflavin (B_2)	2.0 mg.
Niacin	20 mg.
Vitamin B_6	2.5 mg.
Folic Acid	0.8 mcg.
Vitamin B_{12}	8 mcg.
Vitamin C	60 mg.
Vitamin D	400 I.U.
Vitamin E	30 I.U.
Calcium	1,300 mg.
Iron	18 mg.
Magnesium	450 mg.
Zinc	15 mg.
Copper	2 mg.
Biotin	0.3 mg.
Pantothenic acid	10 mg.
Phosphorus	1,300 mg.
Iodine	150 mcg.

GLOSSARY

amniocentesis A test done in the fourth month of pregnancy to detect fetal genetic defects. A long needle is inserted through the mother's abdominal wall, and amniotic fluid is extracted.

Braxton-Hicks contractions Intermittent, usually painless contractions of the uterus that help prepare the organ for pregnancy and labor.

catecholamines Compounds of this class, norepinephrine and epinephrine (adrenaline), are responsible for the "fight or flight" response to stress. High levels of these compounds can adversely affect the developing fetus and inhibit the release of hormones necessary for labor.

colostrum A thin, yellow fluid that is the first milklike food secreted by the breasts, up to a few days after labor.

dilation Opening or widening of the cervix prior to or during labor.

edema Abnormal swelling of the extremities from excess fluid accumulation and retention.

effacement   Thinning of the cervix prior to or during labor.

effleurage   The long, gliding, introductory Swedish massage stroke.

emmenagogue   Herbs pertaining to the female reproductive system.

engagement   The baby dropping into the birth canal.

episiotomy   A surgical incision on the perineum to provide more space for the baby's crowning head.

estrogen   The female sex hormone.

friction   The cross fiber or circular Swedish massage stroke that breaks up muscle spasms and adhesions.

hemoglobin   The protein in blood that gives it color and transports iron.

in utero   Within the uterus (womb).

involution   The uterus returning to its prepregnant condition.

keloid scar   Thick, ropy, discolored scar tissue.

lactation   The process of breast milk production.

lanugo   The hairy coating of the fetus in the fifth and sixth months. A trace may remain on a newborn baby.

lightening   The dropping of the uterus into the pelvis as labor commences.

lochia The normal discharge of blood and mucus from the uterus following birth.

mastitis Inflammation of the breast.

multipara A woman with prior births.

oxytocin The pituitary-produced hormone that stimulates uterine contractions and controls bleeding after birth.

perineum The area between the vagina and the anus.

petrissage The Swedish massage stroke wherein muscle crosses over bone. It is also known as kneading, and it is responsible for increasing muscle tone.

placenta The structure in the uterus where the fetus gets its nourishment.

primapara A woman having her first baby.

progesterone The hormone that prepares the uterus for implantation of the fertilized egg.

prolactin The hormone that stimulates milk production.

quickening The first fetal movements felt by the expectant mother. They are usually felt between the sixteenth and twentieth weeks of pregnancy.

relaxin The hormone responsible for the relaxation of the pelvic ligaments and joints during labor.

sciatica Inflammation of the sciatic nerve. The pain generally courses from the lower back down the middle of the back of one leg.

tapotement A percussive Swedish massage stroke that is stimulatory within the first ten seconds of application and sedative after ten seconds.

toxemia Poisoning during pregnancy. The symptoms are edema, excessive protein in the urine, high blood pressure, rapid weight gain, headaches, and blurring vision. Medical attention is necessary.

vernix caseosa The white, fatty substance covering the newborn's skin.

BIBLIOGRAPHY

Bauer, Cathryn. *Acupressure for Women*. Freedom, Calif.: The Crossing Press, 1987.

Birch, Elizabeth R. "The Experience of Touch Received During Labor." *The Journal of Nurse-Midwifery*, Vol. 31, No. 6 (November/December 1986).

Cain, Kathy. *Partners in Birth*. New York: Warner Books, 1990.

Carter, Mildred. *Hand Reflexology: Key to Perfect Health*. West Nyack, N.Y.: Parker Publishing Company, 1975.

Coalition for the Medical Rights of Women. *Safe Natural Remedies for Discomforts of Pregnancy*. San Francisco, Calif.: Coalition for the Medical Rights of Women, 1981.

Cogan, R. "Postpartum Depression." *ICEA Review*, Vol. 4, No. 2 (August 1980).

Cox, Janice. "Maternal Nutrition During Lactation." *ICEA Review*, Vol. 11, No. 2 (August 1987).

Donsbach, Kurt W. *What You Always Wanted to Know About Pregnancy*. Huntington Beach, Calif.: The International Institute of Natural Health Sciences, 1981.

Fleming, Elise, MA, CCE. *Prenatal Perineal Massage*. Minneapolis, Minn.: ICEA, 1979.

Gardner, Joy. *Healing Yourself During Pregnancy*. Freedom, Calif.: The Crossing Press, 1987.

Goldbeck, Nikki. *As You Eat So Your Baby Grows*. Woodstock, N.Y.: Ceres Press, 1978.

Goldsmith, Judith. *Childbirth Wisdom*. New York: Congdon & Weed, 1984.

Haire, Doris. *How the Breast Functions*. Minneapolis, Minn.: ICEA, 1970.

Hazle, Nancy R. "Postpartum Blues—Assessment and Intervention." *The Journal of Nurse-Midwifery*, Vol. 27, No. 6 (November/December 1982).

Inkeles, Gordon. *Massage and Peaceful Pregnancy*. New York: Putnam Publishing Group, 1983.

Jiménez, Sherry. *The Pregnant Woman's Comfort Guide*. Englewood Cliffs, N.J.: Prentice-Hall, 1983.

Jones, Carl. *The Birth Partner's Handbook*. New York: Meadowbrook Press, 1989.

Kunz, Barbara and Kevin. *The Complete Guide to Foot Reflexology*. Albuquerque, N.M.: Reflexology Research Project, 1980.

Lawrence, Mary Ellen. "How to Massage a Pregnant Lady." *Well-Being*, No. 46, pp. 27–32.

Leboyer, Frederick. *Loving Hands*. New York: Alfred A. Knopf, Inc., 1976.

Malstrom, Stan. *Natural Approach to Female Problems*. Orem, Ut.: BiWorld Publishers, 1982.

McCarthy, Paul. "Getting Baby Born on Time." *American Health* (October 1985).

McKay, S. "Maternal Stress and Pregnancy Outcome." *ICEA Review*, Vol. 4, No. 1 (April 1980).

Parks, Gael. "Massage Therapy for Women." *Well-Being*, No. 24 (September 1977).

Schrag, Kathryn. "Maintenance of Pelvic Floor Integrity During Childbirth." *The Journal of Nurse-Midwifery*, Vol. 24, No. 6 (November/December 1979).

"Supplements and Common Sense." *Prevention* (May 1986).

Tisserand, Maggie. *Aromatherapy for Women*. New York: Thorsons Publishers, 1985.

Todd, Linda. *Labor and Birth Guide for You*. Minneapolis, Minn.: ICEA, 1981.

U.S. Department of Health and Human Services. *Prenatal and*

Postnatal Care. Wilmington, Del.: Stuart Pharmaceuticals, 1981.

Verrilli, George E., and Anne Marie Mueser. *While Waiting*. New York: St. Martin's Press, 1982.

WGBH Education Foundation. *The Miracle of Life*. Boston, Mass.: *Nova*, 1983.

Yates, John. *A Physician's Guide to Therapeutic Massage*. Vancouver, B.C.: Massage Therapists' Association of British Columbia, 1990.

Young, Diony. *Bonding—How Parents Become Attached to Their Baby*. Minneapolis, Minn.: ICEA, 1978.

INDEX

161